THE DOCTORS WE NEED

Imagining a New Path for Physician Recruitment, Training, and Support

ANTHONY SANFILIPPO

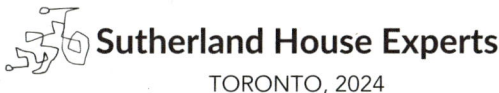

Sutherland House Experts

TORONTO, 2024

Sutherland House Experts Corporation
260 Heath Street West
Suite 605
Toronto, Ontario
M5P 3L6

Copyright © 2024 by Anthony Sanfilippo

All rights reserved, including the right to reproduce this book or portions thereof in any form whatsoever. For information on rights and permissions or to request a special discount for bulk purchases, please contact Sutherland House Experts at info@sutherlandhouseexperts.com

Sutherland House Experts and logo are registered trademarks.

First edition, November 2024

Manufactured in Turkey
Cover designed by Jordan Lunn
Cover images courtesy of Freepik

Library and Archives Canada Cataloguing in Publication
Title: The doctors we need : imagining a new path for physician recruitment, training, and support / Anthony Sanfilippo.
Names: Sanfilippo, Anthony, author.
Description: Includes bibliographical references.
Identifiers: Canadiana (print) 20240460901 | Canadiana (ebook) 20240461037 | ISBN 9781738396467 (hardcover) | ISBN 9781738396474 (EPUB)
Subjects: LCSH: Physicians (General practice)—Supply and demand—Canada. | LCSH: Physicians (General practice)—Recruiting—Canada. | LCSH: Medical education—Canada. | LCSH: Health care reform—Canada. | LCSH: Primary care (Medicine)—Canada. | LCSH: Family medicine—Canada.
Classification: LCC RA410.9.C2 S26 2024 | DDC 362.10971—dc23

ISBN 978-1-7383964-6-7
eBook 978-1-7383964-7-4

More Praise for Sanfilippo's *The Doctors We Need*

"This warmly written, story-rich book explores the widening chasm between society's primary care needs and our archaic structures of medical education and practice. Dr. Sanfilippo's diagnosis and remedies are sensible, thoughtful and long overdue."
—Dr. David Walker, Former Dean of Queen's Medical School

"Through story-telling and thoughtful analysis, *The Doctors We Need* traces the 'family doctor crisis' to its roots in medical education. Sanfilippo is uniquely qualified to suggest a remedy for this malady, and his prescription is bold and creative. If implemented, it would fundamentally change how we choose and train doctors and shake up our primary healthcare system to its very core."
—Richard K. Reznick, OC, MD, FRCSC, FACS, FRCSEd (hon), FRCSI (hon), FRCS (hon), Professor Emeritus of Surgery and Dean Emeritus, Queen's University and Past President Royal College of Physicians and Surgeons of Canada

"Dr. Sanfilippo unpacks a complex problem facing many Canadians: a lack of access to family physicians and timely primary care. He does this in a way that every reader can understand, no matter their background. His proposed solutions are innovative, thoughtful, and achievable!"
—Dr. Tony Stone, Family Physician, and educator of family physicians

"Dr. S has created an accurate and on-point explanation for our present primary care crisis that starts with stories where physicians and patients will see themselves portrayed, continues with demystifying the complex medical education system, and finishes with clear-headed solutions."

—Bruce Wright MD CCFP FCFP, Regional Associate Dean of the Island Medical Program at UBC, Head and Professor of Division of Medical Sciences at the University of Victoria, and former President of the Medical Council of Canada

"A rare insider's look at medical education in Canada from one of the country's most respected leaders in medical pedagogy. Inspiring, credible and highly pragmatic solutions to vexing issues at a time when most others are only able to eloquently describe the problem. A must-read for all who care about the future of the MD workforce in Canada."

—Chris Simpson MD, Former President of the Canadian Medical Association (2014–2015) and Professor in the Department of Medicine at Queen's University

"Dr. Anthony Sanfilippo, through compelling patient stories, powerfully illustrates the horrific consequences of Canadians' inability to access foundational primary care. These narratives reveal the profound impacts on patients and their families, clinicians, the overall healthcare system, our economy, and society at large. His solution? Integrated primary care teams delivering patient-centered care, reforming policy of admission to medical school and curricular reform, all in order to attract top clinicians to practice family medicine. With a focus on funding improved health outcomes over the outdated fee-for-service structure, 'The Doctors We Need' asks: Can we achieve this critical transformation?"

—Professor Colleen M. Flood, Dean of Queen's University Faculty of Law

The Doctors We Need

To my parents, John and Grace, who encouraged my pursuit of medical school and worked to get me there, and to my wife Michelle, whose love and support got me through it.

"And who is my neighbor?"

Luke 10:29

EDITORIAL NOTE

IT'S IMPORTANT TO CLARIFY TERMINOLOGY. The terms *primary care, general practice, family physician*, and *family medicine* have all been used somewhat interchangeably but all have specific meanings.

Primary care refers to the provision of integrated, accessible health care services that could be termed both comprehensive and continuing. It is intended to achieve both better health and better care. Primary care is usually provided by physicians, but can also be provided by other health professionals, such as nurse practitioners, or in the context of integrated teams.

General Practice is now a somewhat antiquated term that had been used to describe physicians practicing without a particular specialty focus. At one point, all physicians graduated as "General Practitioners." As we'll learn, this is no longer the case.

Family Medicine is now a separate specialty within medical practice with its own training program and certifying college. Family Medicine doctors (*family physicians*) provide primary care, as well as other services related to their specialty. Their goals are best described in the professional profile provided by the Canadian College of Family Physicians.[1]

---

[1] College of Family Physicians of Canada. (n.d.). *Family medicine professional profile*. Retrieved from https://www.cfpc.ca/CFPC/media/Resources/Education/FM-Professional-Profile.pdf

Working together, family physicians provide a system of front-line health care that is accessible, high-quality, comprehensive, and continuous. Individually they take responsibility for the overarching and proactive medical care of patients, ensuring follow-up and facilitating transitions of care and/or referrals when required. More than a series of tasks, it is through relational continuity and a commitment to a broad scope of practice that the complexity of care is meaningfully addressed. The care family physicians provide improves the overall health of the population.

In the United States, the terminology and scope of practice for family medicine is broadly similar to Canada. Family medicine is recognized as a distinct medical specialty focused on comprehensive primary care across all ages and stages of life. The American Academy of Family Physicians (AAFP) defines family medicine as "*the medical specialty which provides continuing, comprehensive health care for the individual and family. It is a specialty in breadth that integrates the biological, clinical and behavioral sciences.*" Family physicians in the United States complete a 3-year residency training program after medical school to become board-certified. Their training encompasses all aspects of primary care, including pediatrics, obstetrics, internal medicine, and surgery.

In keeping with this definition and the intention of this book to focus on provision of primary care specifically by physicians, the terms *family physician (or family doctor)* and *family practice* will be used throughout.

The accounts contained in the book are based on real medical encounters but have been altered to emphasize key points and protect the identity of the individuals involved.

CONTENTS

Dedication	vii
Quotation	ix
Editorial Note	xi
Introduction: The Dilemma	1
Chapter 1: Sara's Story	7
Chapter 2: Rachel's Story	17
Chapter 3: What We Expect of Our Doctors	24
Chapter 4: The Contemporary Physician	32
Chapter 5: Out of One, Many	46
Chapter 6: The Challenges of Generalism	63
Chapter 7: The Elephant in the Room	75
Chapter 8: Who Becomes a Doctor?	83
Chapter 9: The Long, Narrow Path	100
Chapter 10: Who's Driving the Bus?	106
Chapter 11: Failing to Deliver	116

Chapter 12: *Disruptive Innovation 1:* Connecting Medical
School Admissions to Societal Needs 129

Chapter 13: *Disruptive Innovation 2:* Connecting Medical
Education to Societal Needs 137

Chapter 14: Is Disruptive Innovation Realistic Within
Medical Education? 142

Chapter 15: *Disruptive Innovation 3:* Restructure Care
Delivery to Better Meet Patient and
Physician Needs 144

Chapter 16: Can We Change? 157

Acknowledgements 160

References 163

INTRODUCTION

The Dilemma

*S*ARA HAS RECENTLY BEEN DISCHARGED *from hospital after several weeks in Intensive Care, where she was treated for an illness that could have been prevented if she had a family doctor. She's now home but, still without a family doctor, she doesn't know where to turn for follow-up care and medication adjustments.*

Brandon is two weeks old. Because his parents are without a family doctor, so is he. His first-time parents have questions about his care. Why is he crying so much? Does he need immunizations?

Sharon has found a breast lump on self-examination. She's scared and not sure what to do. The family doctor she's known since childhood retired a few months ago.

Joel is a 35-year-old computer programmer who has had mental health problems and needs his medications prescribed. The doctor who's been providing counseling and prescribing his medications has retired and was unable to find a replacement.

Nicole has recently moved to a large city, living on her own. She's been on a waiting list for a family doctor but has been told there are thousands of others in the same situation. She's been having unusual bleeding and not sure what to do.

These are real people, living among us, today. They are a sampling of about six million of our fellow Canadians, a number that is surely growing.

In response, and in desperation, mayors and elected officials are meeting in towns and cities across our country to develop strategies to attract and retain doctors to their communities. In doing so, they are competing with each other for a limited resource, the source of which they cannot address or influence.

All this is happening in a country that purports to provide universal access to health care for all its citizens and has a highly respected medical community and processes for training them that are sources of pride and distinction.

How does this happen?

To put this into focus, let's consider three contemporary realities.

Canadian society values universal and comprehensive health care for all its citizens as a fundamental right.

In our country, this is not simply a lofty aspiration or "nice to have some day" idea. It is a contemporary expectation of all citizens and is assured by our government. Legally, it's established in the *Canada Health Act* which is in place "to protect, promote and restore the physical and mental well-being of residents of Canada and to facilitate reasonable access to health services without financial barriers."[2] It is therefore a commitment. Moreover, most would see it as a defining characteristic of the sort of caring and compassionate society we aspire to be, and which, we expect, sets Canada apart as an example for others to emulate.

Admittedly, when the concept of universal health care was initially envisioned and accepted, expectations were more modest than they

---

[2] Health Canada. (n.d.). *Canada Health Act*. Government of Canada. Retrieved from https://www.canada.ca/en/health-canada/services/health-care-system/canada-health-care-system-medicare/canada-health-act.html

are today. A commitment that grew out of a desire to ensure everyone had access to lifesaving care when needed has expanded far beyond "illness care" to encompass a broader vision of "health" that aims to prevent those life-threatening illnesses from ever happening, promote general well-being, and optimize functionality at all stages of life. Despite that expanding expectation, the commitment has never been seriously challenged and remains very much in place.

The second reality is that, **for most Canadians, *access to health care (particularly in its broader sense) requires the assistance and guidance of a professional provider.*** That person has been, since the notion of universal health care came into being several decades ago, a primary care physician. In the past, that person was not only the point of *access* but also the primary *provider* of most care. Every Canadian had, or could have, such a person in their lives. At one point, when they all basically did the same job, they were simply "doctors." As specialties began to emerge, they became known as "general practitioners" to differentiate them from doctors who limited their work to specific illnesses or procedures. For the past few decades, they've become known as "family physicians" and are considered a specialty that provides the *comprehensive* and *continuing* care essential to ensuring access and maintenance of health. In short, the promise of universal accessible health care is simply not possible without that primary point of contact. Lack of a family doctor significantly impedes access to timely help.

Reality Three is that, **according to the most recent information, *15% of Canadians report having no affiliation with a family doctor.*** [3] That amounts to about six million people, a figure that is expected to increase in coming years.

---

[3] Statistics Canada. (n.d.). *Table 13-10-0484-01 Life expectancy and other elements of the life table, Canada, all provinces except Prince Edward Island.* Retrieved from https://doi.org/10.25318/1310048401-eng

And so, our three realities lead to the conclusion that the common goals of the medical profession and our national and provincial governments to provide for the health care needs of all citizens are not being met. A trust, a covenant, has been breached.

That realization should also cause us to explore some key questions:

1. Does it even matter? Are we actually worse off, or are we simply seeing a natural evolution that we've not yet come to grips with?
2. Why? How has it come to be? What are the root causes?
3. Can anything be done about it, or is this simply a new reality that will have to be accepted with adjustment in our expectations?

In the chapters that follow we will explore each of these themes. We'll do so by encountering real-life folks, both patients and doctors, who are directly involved.

In the first two chapters, we'll explore the impact of the doctor shortage by reviewing and examining the lived experiences of patients and physicians who have been impacted.

In the chapters that follow, we'll go back to basics to explore underlying causes and their role in the family medicine crisis that we're facing. Using real life accounts, we'll explore:

- Our evolving expectations of what our doctors should be doing for us.
- How contemporary doctors have expectations of themselves and their professional obligations that are not always aligned with societal expectations.
- How the nature of medical practice has evolved such that a huge diversity of roles is required, and the people filling those roles must be similarly diverse with respect to their skills and interests.

- How the concept of the generalist doctor, so essential to family medicine and primary care, differs from other more focused areas of medicine, and brings with it particular challenges.
- How the ways we compensate doctors for their work disadvantages primary care and undermines the value of their work.
- How the process by which we admit people to medical school fails to target attributes, interests, and commitment relevant to primary care.
- How our long-established medical education processes have failed to adapt to the changes in medical practice and are both lengthening training times for all specialties and disadvantaging family practice in particular.
- How decision-making and substantive reform are hampered by the multiple and independent institutions and entities involved in various aspects of the medical education process.

We'll find ourselves drawn to some important conclusions:

The medical needs of our society have exploded. Advances in medical care have been staggeringly successful in reducing the burden of disease and allowing us to live longer and more active lives.

With those changes, the medical profession has also changed. No longer can a single doctor provide all aspects of care that a patient might require over the course of their life. No longer is medicine an independent undertaking pursued by people of a homogeneous type. The very term "medical doctor" applies to well over a hundred different specialties and areas of interest. The family physician, who provides "comprehensive and continuing care" to patients over their lifetime, has become one of those hyper-specialties.

We have not adapted to those changes. The processes by which we select, train, and support doctors remain rooted in the same institutional and regulatory structures and have not fully adapted to changing needs. It is not the 1970s anymore, or even the early aughts.

We strangely lack the collective will and means to adapt—and this is unacceptable. Despite a large number of institutions, colleges and professional organizations involved in these processes, we lack the ability to enact effective change. Canada needs to do better and the medical profession has both the knowledge and responsibility to promote needed reform.

We'll then bring together the various themes and attempt to develop some key interventions that have potential to address the problem.

We will find that we are, in fact, facing what the late Clayton Christensen described as *"The Innovator's Dilemma"*—an unwillingness to abandon traditional and previously successful practices. Failures of large and previously flourishing businesses and industries can be traced to an unwillingness to acknowledge that the tried and true was no longer addressing the evolving needs of their markets. Recognizing the need to change is, of course, only part of the formula for ongoing success. The courage to change in the face of seeming continuing productivity is essential, and exceedingly difficult to engage, particularly in the absence of a clear, centralized authority. Without it, we are leaving mayors and town councils to assist their constituents with whatever means are available to them.

What might that change look like? To begin, let's start by looking a little more closely at one of the folks affected by all this. Her story, and that of the doctors she's encountered along the way will help us better understand the roots of our dilemma and perhaps provide insights to potential solutions.

And so, let's start by meeting the aforementioned Sara…

CHAPTER ONE

Sara's Story

MEET SARA. SHE IS A 65-year-old woman who, together with her husband, immigrated to Canada over four decades ago. They settled in a small city where they joined a community of people of their own cultural background and language. They worked in a variety of service jobs until saving enough money to open a small convenience store which they still operate, seven days a week, doing most of the work themselves. They have raised four children, who, over the years, have worked in the store after hours and on weekends. All four children earned university degrees and are now thriving in their various careers.

Sara has always enjoyed good health but has been feeling unwell for the past several weeks. Known for her prodigious stamina and work ethic, Sara is now much more tired and finding it distressingly difficult to get through her daily activities. Always an excellent cook who enjoyed large family meals, she now feels that her appetite seems to have abandoned her. She has been feverish at night, sometimes waking drenched in sweat. More recently, she has been more breathless doing her usual work in the home and in the store.

Sara has no family physician. The doctor she and her husband had seen for many years retired several years ago and, despite multiple attempts, they've not been able to find a replacement. Since feeling unwell, she's taken some home remedies suggested by friends in her community. She's visited a walk-in clinic twice and, each time, was given courses of antibiotics. Nothing has helped. In fact, her symptoms have escalated. She finds she has to stop to catch her breath after doing things that came easily to her even a few weeks ago, such as retrieving something from the basement.

At the insistence of her husband and one of her daughters, she returns to the walk-in clinic. There, she's seen by a young physician she's meeting for the first time. The doctor listens to her account of the illness, sees the concern on the part of her family members, and notes the previous courses of antibiotics that have not been helpful. The doctor also recognizes that Sara simply doesn't look well and has the strong impression that she is not someone who is likely to complain or seek help for a trivial issue. On examination, Sara's blood pressure is a little low and her heart rate high. The doctor examines Sara's mouth and eyes, looks closely at her hands and nails, and listens to her heart and lungs. Sara seems anemic and has a heart murmur. The cause of the murmur isn't clear, but it sounds alarming.

Based on all this, the doctor isn't sure of the diagnosis but suspects a very serious cardiac condition or infection and feels Sara requires urgent assessment. Blood work and cultures are ordered, which can be carried out at the clinic, and a requisition is completed for an echocardiogram (ultrasound of the heart), but the doctor knows that will likely take a few weeks.

So, what to do? Sara's condition requires urgent assessment, but it isn't really an emergency, and the doctor is very much aware of how busy the local emergency department is with life-threatening problems and patients waiting many hours just to be seen. Who will follow up on the results of the blood work? The doctor isn't scheduled to do another walk-in clinic shift for several weeks and isn't even sure whether she's in a position to receive the results of the tests that have just been arranged. And, by the way, there are another fifteen patients waiting to be seen.

The doctor decides to have Sara and her family go home after the blood work but gets her phone number and tells them to await further instructions. After a long day of work at the clinic, the doctor gets on the phone and begins to call the hospital switchboard with requests to be connected to several specialist services to identify one that will see Sara urgently. Most indicate that they are "on-call" only for emergencies and that a consultation request should be sent to their departmental office. Most wait times are measured in months. With much pleading, one finally agrees to see Sara in two days in an "urgent clinic." All this has taken several calls, multiple repetitions of the story, plus a few hours, now well into the evening.

When Sara is seen in that clinic, the blood work that the walk-in clinic doctor ordered indicates that an infectious process is underway as manifest by high white blood cell counts, low hemoglobin, signs of renal injury, active infection, and blood cultures positive for a species of staphylococccal bacteria. The now urgently arranged echocardiogram shows that Sara has a congenitally abnormal (bicuspid) aortic valve and aneurysm (dangerous enlargement) of her aorta. The valve has become infected. She has endocarditis, which is considered a medical emergency. She is immediately admitted to hospital under an internal medicine "admitting service."

Over the next several weeks in hospital, she is treated with high doses of intravenous antibiotics.

She requires insertion of an indwelling catheter to receive the antibiotics.

She develops *C. difficile* secondary to the antibiotics and requires treatment under isolation, which means her family can't visit.

She has a "ministroke" due to an embolism from the infected valve and requires several CT and MRI scans as she (very fortunately) recovers neurologically.

Despite the antibiotics, the infection doesn't resolve, and follow-up echocardiograms show that the infection is progressing. It is decided that she must undergo surgical replacement of her aortic valve and repair of the aneurysm.

It is a long and complicated operation carried out by two cardiac surgeons and specialized cardiac anesthesiologists.

Post-operatively, she develops pulmonary infections that require prolonged intubation (mechanically assisted breathing) and further courses of antibiotics.

She develops renal failure and must undergo dialysis.

She develops heart block (a dangerous slowing of her heart rate) and requires a pacemaker.

She has episodes of atrial fibrillation (an abnormal acceleration of heart rhythm) requiring cardioversion (re-establishment of regular rhythm using a therapeutic does of electric current delivered to the heart and intravenous medications).

After three weeks on the cardiology ward and ten weeks in ICU, she has recovered sufficiently to be transferred to a rehabilitation service at another hospital to complete her recovery and receive physio- and occupational therapy.

Finally, Sara is fully recovered and ready to go home, but before that, she has been treated by:

- General internists
- Cardiologists
- Infectious disease specialists
- Laboratory medicine specialists
- Cardiac surgeons
- Interventional cardiologists
- Interventional radiologists

- Neurologists
- Gastroenterologists
- Nephrologists
- Vascular surgeons
- Intensive care physicians
- Rehabilitation medicine specialists

She has also benefited from the care of dozens of specialized nurses, therapists, and laboratory staff. She has, by all accounts, received exemplary care that has been lifesaving. Everyone involved has entered her care at a point at which Sara's needs and their expertise and skills intersected. They provided excellent care and, when the need for their care had resolved, the specialists disengaged.

And now, Sara is ready to return home. But she still has no family doctor. There is no one outside the hospital system to take up her care, which is now quite complicated. At a follow-up visit at the pacemaker clinic for a routine check, she and her family ask the nurses and cardiologists a few very practical questions.

- She's been discharged on a long list of medications and isn't sure about their purpose or which are to be maintained. And for how long? Who will reassess and re-prescribe?
- She's having difficulty sleeping and concentrating. Why? Will this resolve?
- Can she return to work in the store? Her husband is having difficulty coping alone.
- Sara herself asks whether her children might have the same cardiac condition as she does (which they may). This has not been raised previously. Who will help them resolve this?

Sara's long-term success will not be determined by any of the people who were involved in her long hospitalization, but by whoever oversees her ongoing care. Like over six million other Canadians, Sara has no such individual to whom she can turn.

The Consequences of Not Having a Family Doctor

Sara's story highlights many important implications.

<u>Delayed Diagnosis</u>. Access to a family doctor familiar with her background and personality would likely have led to an earlier diagnosis and, potentially, a less advanced disease and less complicated course after the diagnosis was finally made. The family doctor would have followed up on the initial antibiotic attempts and recognized sooner that she was not responding.

<u>Awareness of Risk</u>. Sara's congenital valve disease put her at high risk for endocarditis in the context of any infection. It's likely that a family doctor, having had the opportunity to meet and examine Sara previously, would have been aware that she had longstanding valve disease and would have had an increased awareness of the implications of a continuing infection.

<u>Continuing Care</u>. Sara's need for care does not end with her discharge from hospital. In fact, in many ways, it's just the beginning. The practical concerns she brought to her pacemaker clinic appointment are important and, although not immediately life threatening, will go a long way to determining her recovery and the likelihood of having a recurrence. For most patients, it's their family physician who provides or oversees that continuing convalescent care.

<u>Prevention</u>. Subsequent episodes of endocarditis can be prevented with the judicious use of antibiotics in certain situations. A family physician, aware of her history, will be able to recognize such situations and provide appropriate prophylactic care. In addition, ongoing control of her blood pressure, glucose levels, weight, and levels of exercise will all be important to her ongoing health.

Compliance. Sara is much more likely to accept and carry out treatment recommendations if she's dealing with someone she knows and trusts. That trust is much more likely to develop in a continuing relationship, such as she would develop with an empathetic and approachable family physician.

Excess Use of Emergency Departments. Although Sara chose to initially go to an urgent care center, many patients who lack a family physician are feeling the need to go to emergency departments with similar or even less serious issues. They are not to blame for this. Without the ability to get medical advice in other ways, they can't be expected to judge the urgency of the problems they're experiencing.

Delayed Hospital Discharges. Without a family physician to assume post-discharge care, to ensure they are safe and receiving appropriate care, patients are being kept in hospital longer than would otherwise have been required.

Longer Wait Times for Procedural Care. More advanced disease at presentation increases the need for diagnostic and therapeutic procedures, increasing wait times for all.

And, finally, all these consequences lead to *increased costs* for an already strained health care system. If every patient without a family physician requires even three avoidable and unscheduled encounters with the health care system a year, this amounts to 18 million additional visits, most of which will occur in after-hours clinics or emergency departments.

As we learned earlier, Sara is far from alone. Not all will be unfortunate enough to experience the sort of illness she has, but all are at risk. Consider a few more examples.

Amanda, Craig, and Brandon

Amanda and Craig have been eagerly anticipating the birth of their first child. Although they don't have a family doctor, they have been able to get advice from family and friends, have access to much online information, and have been able to join prenatal classes at the local health unit. They purchase a blood pressure kit to monitor Amanda's blood pressure during the pregnancy because there is a history of such problems in her family. They even purchase some urine test strips and research how to use them and interpret the results. Fortunately, the pregnancy goes well. When the time comes for delivery, they report to the local hospital and, after a long but uncomplicated delivery, Brandon comes into their lives, a healthy seven-and-a-half-pound baby boy. They get great care from the nurses and doctors staffing the labor and delivery floor, and next day, as she's recovering and being prepared for discharge, Amanda is asked by the nursing staff who will be Brandon's family doctor. The hospital is preparing Brandon's records and would like to send them along to whoever will be assuming his care.

Brandon, of course, has no family doctor. This is because his parents have no family doctor. And they do require care. Although Brandon appears to be a healthy baby, he will almost certainly come down with various ailments and infections common to infants and young children. He will require immunizations, and it's known that periodic checks to screen for problems and ensure development is progressing normally can be very effective in preventing serious illness and promoting health. It's also likely that Amanda and Craig, as first-time parents, will require some counseling and support as they take on their new roles as parents.

Sharon is a 29-year-old single woman who has a family history of breast cancer. As a result, she examines herself regularly. One morning she feels an area of firmness in her left breast that seems new to her. She's very concerned and not sure what to do next. Is this an emergency?

Joel is a 35-year-old computer programmer who has had mental health problems since his youth. For many years, he's been doing well on a complex list of medications and regular check-ups and review with his family doctor who he trusts and relies upon. That doctor is retiring, and Joel has been unable to find a replacement. Joel doesn't know who to turn to or even how to get his medications renewed when his current supply finishes.

What's required to address all this?

Given that the case load for family physicians averages about 1,500 patients, about 4,000 new doctors would be required to accommodate those 6 million people.

Now let's examine the pipeline. Our seventeen (soon to be twenty) Canadian medical schools graduate approximately 3,000 new doctors each year. But these graduates are not yet ready for practice. They will all require further training and select between about thirty "entry-level" specialties. Most specialize further in future years into over 100 discrete specialties, subspecialties, and sub-subspecialties.

Only about 40 percent choose to engage in family medicine as a career, and about 50 percent of those are opting to provide that continuing, comprehensive care that would address the needs of those unattached patients. Simple arithmetic tells us that the current pipeline will result in no more than about 700 additional family doctors each year.

And the problem isn't likely to improve soon. One in six of the 47,000 or so family doctors currently practicing in Canada are at or beyond retirement age. Moreover, the problem isn't limited to family medicine. Many other much needed specialties are experiencing similar shortfalls, including, to name a few, psychiatry, pediatrics, oncology and pathology.

How did we get to such a desperate state? As we'll see, our current crisis is the result of the natural evolution and expansion of health care that has occurred over the past several decades. That growth, although welcome and beneficial in many ways, has not been met with appropriate responses in how we select, train, or support physicians. We'll explore these issues in upcoming chapters. But, before doing so, it's important to examine the other side of this dilemma—the doctors who are attempting to provide much needed primary care. Their experience is as important as that of the Saras among us in understanding those root causes.

So, let's meet the doctor who assessed Sara initially in the walk-in clinic and got the whole process underway—Rachel.

CHAPTER TWO

Rachel's Story

SARA HAS SURVIVED A DEVASTING illness that would have certainly taken her life if not for the efforts and skills of many very well-trained physicians and health care providers. It is, by any measure, a successful outcome and illustration of what modern medical care can accomplish. But none of this would have happened if not for the efforts of that primary care physician in the walk-in clinic who took the time to listen, recognized the severity of Sara's illness, and undertook extraordinary efforts to get her seen urgently.

That person may be unknown to anyone else involved in Sara's care, even to Sara herself. That person may not even be aware of the events that transpired after the initial referral. That person was almost certainly the least well compensated of any individual involved in Sara's care and has to spend a hefty portion of her pay on administrative staff and overhead, as would any small businessperson.

That person is Rachel. She was raised in a small Ontario community. Her father is a pharmacist, and her mother a retired elementary school teacher. Rachel grew up watching and getting to know the various doctors in the community who depended on her father to fill prescriptions for their patients. She saw how they cared for the needs of people throughout their lives and in the context of whatever problems they developed. Rachel decided from an early age that she wanted to become that sort of doctor and return to her home community to practice.

A bright and eager student, Rachel excelled in her studies and obtained a university scholarship. One of the happiest days of her life was when she was accepted into medical school at a prestigious Ontario university. She embraced her studies with the knowledge that she was preparing for her life's work and graduated with distinction, entering a residency in family medicine. After 2 years in that training program, she returned to her community to take up the practice she'd always dreamed of.

But things were not as she'd imagined.

Her training enabled her to diagnose most issues that her patients developed, but many required much more sophisticated testing than could be provided in her office or nearby lab and had to be arranged and scheduled at teaching hospitals some distance away. That scheduling differed for every test and every site. Just keeping track of how to get a particular test carried out was a challenge. Once scheduled, wait times were long and she worried constantly about patients getting more seriously ill while waiting for a definitive diagnosis.

Many patients required the involvement of another specialist of some type. Most often, these were not available in her community and had to be arranged and scheduled. Again, the arrangements were different for every specialty. In fact, for every specialist! Once in place, wait times were often much longer than she was comfortable with, and she found herself again worrying about her patient's condition while they'd be waiting for care. Often, she would try to call a consultant directly to get advice or advocate for an earlier assessment.

Arranging those calls was also very difficult, and she was often made to feel like she was bothering them unnecessarily.

She was finding that the electronic medical record (EMR) system her office was using demanded much of her time. She was required to enter not only her findings and recommendations, but also many other aspects of the encounter. She was finding that the need to complete the EMR was taking time away from speaking with patients and understanding the nature of their medical challenges. On top of that, she was left with much to complete at the end of her day, often requiring her to work late into the night.

Her practice grew quickly. She was continually being asked to take on new patients in the community who were without a family doctor. She obliged at first but gradually found she was unable to book appointments in what she considered a reasonable time and so, painfully, had to close her practice to new patients. The requests did not stop and were getting increasingly desperate. Comments in the media from the public, the government, and even from other doctors implied that the problem was simply that she and other family doctors like her weren't working hard enough! She knew it wasn't true and that she shouldn't take it seriously, but she found such commentary hurtful and discouraging.

She was finding that her work was wreaking serious impositions on her personal life. She'd met Daniel in university. They got married after he completed his engineering degree. They were planning to have children, and Rachel had been trying to arrange a maternity leave for about a year but, despite there being another ten physicians in her Family Health Team, no one could take on her patients and she'd been unable to find a replacement.

Perhaps most troubling of all, Rachel was finding that the reality and expectations of medical practice were at odds with her personal goals and basic principles she'd embraced through her training. Throughout medical school and residency, the principle of work–life balance had been emphasized. The fundamental concept was that it was critical to ensure that doctors ensure they had time in their lives for personal pursuits and time away from the rigors of medical practice. This was fundamental to their personal wellness, both physical and mental. It was also considered essential to their ability to continue to function effectively, maintain competence, and minimize errors. In other words, a healthy work–life balance was something that would protect themselves, their families, and their patients, too. This principle was applied in the scheduling of their classes in medical school and further enforced through regulations that governed the number of hours she could be on call and mandatory time off during the work week. All this was supported by medical student societies and, during residency, by professional organizations that negotiated terms of engagement with hospitals and universities in much the same manner as would a labor union, including union-like assertiveness and the threat of strike actions. Accounts of how previous generations of physicians were continually available without such regulations were used as examples of the sort of practice patterns that were counter to the principles of personal wellness and should be eschewed.

But, in practice, Rachel encountered an environment where no such mandated protections were in place. She sensed subtle, unstated expectations from her patients and colleagues that she *should* be available for various clinical and even administrative purposes far beyond the standard work week. There were also expectations from consulting specialists that she be available to discuss or take up aspects of a patient's care regardless of her schedule. She would get referral letters and hospital discharge summaries outlining several "suggestions" or "recommendations" that read like a task list for her, without any prior notification or request. She felt barraged with expectations she could not control and which far exceeded what she had been taught would allow for an appropriate work–life balance. She also felt powerless to do anything about it.

As a result of all this, Rachel decided about a year ago to give up her family medicine practice and start doing locums (temporary roles in different locations, replacing doctors on leave or vacation). She tried for about a year to find someone to take her practice but was unsuccessful. In the end, she simply had to inform her patients of her decision. Many were resentful. Some said they were sad to hear but could understand. This was an excruciating decision and process for her, and she continues to feel guilty about it. But it has allowed her to stay in practice, providing temporary relief to other family physicians, and doing shifts in urgent care centers, like the one where she encountered Sara.

Multiple Victims. Same Cause. Engaging the Problem.

And so, our stories illustrate multiple victims of the same systemic problem. A patient whose care was compromised and who suffered medically because of delayed care that may have been prevented if she'd been able to access a family physician earlier. A highly capable and dedicated doctor who left her practice, at least in part because there were insufficient physicians to share the load. We're aware that there are millions of such people in our country who lack access to a family physician. Counting the number of Rachels is more difficult, but common experience and reports would suggest that the number of doctors leaving family practice that provides comprehensive and continuing care is increasing.

And there are many signs indicating things are likely to get much worse soon. Only about 40 percent of medical students choose to enter family medicine training programs. Of those, almost half elect to undertake practices in areas of focused interest (such as emergency medicine, care of the elderly, palliative care, or sports medicine), or even simply to do temporary assignments (locums) as did Rachel. In other words, the proportion of doctors entering comprehensive family practice is diminishing.

As was pointed out previously, the current medical education "supply chain" is not producing nearly enough doctors to address even the current needs. Our system of recruiting and training doctors is clearly failing, and rather spectacularly so.

Many causes and solutions have been suggested, but these have generally called for expansions in the current processes for educating, training, and recruiting physicians. If we pour in more resources and ramp up the engine, the hope is that we will produce more of the type of doctors we need and are lacking.

In truth, doing more of the same will not resolve this issue—this a feeling shared widely within the medical profession, yet the profession itself has not grappled with this reality. As is always the case with complex problems, effective and durable solutions require deeper understanding of root causes. This is not new thinking. Aristotle spoke of this concept millennia ago:

> *In every systematic inquiry (methodos) where there are first principles, or causes, or elements, knowledge and science result from acquiring knowledge of these.*
>
> —Aristotle, *Physics* (184a10-16)

And so, what are the "first principles" that are relevant to our understanding of this medical care dilemma in which we find ourselves? In considering our approach, we must begin by accepting a difficult and uncomfortable truth: *the process by which we select, educate, and train physicians in Canada is not meeting the needs of our citizens.*

Acceptance of this truth leads us to a need for a thoughtful, candid, and objective dissection and examination of that process, out of which will emerge root causes that can be addressed through directed and targeted solutions.

The next few chapters will begin that dissection, focusing on some fundamental questions.

- What do doctors do?
- What do we need doctors to do?
- How do we select and train doctors?
- How do we engage doctors?
- Who controls these processes?

In doing so, we'll be challenging the traditional and widely accepted practices. We will illustrate with examples and stories drawn from real life and attempt to contrast current realities with needs. It will not be comfortable, but real change requires blunt and objective analysis. We'll conclude in the final chapters with suggestions for radical change based on that analysis.

And so, we begin with a simple question. What do we expect of our doctors?

CHAPTER THREE

What We Expect of Our Doctors

M Y MONDAY MORNING CLINIC IS usually a pretty busy place. In addition to a number of patients I have seen previously and am now reassessing, there are usually three or four "news." These are folks I've never met before, referred from other physicians for assessment of symptoms that may be related to a cardiac problem.

One recent morning, my first "new" was Harry. He's a retired school principal who has been quite healthy and very active throughout his life. He and his wife have been spending their retirement years golfing, visiting grandchildren, and taking cruises. He's eager to tell me that he's been to six of the seven continents and either walks or bicycles at least an hour each day. When we get around to the reason for him being in my clinic, it seems he's been noticing that he's having more difficulty doing a number of things. When I ask for examples, he cites being more breathless after walking the elevations on his golf course and feeling fatigued after helping his grandson move recently. No pain, but definitely breathing harder and more tired the next day. He's been reading up on his symptoms and is concerned this may be an early sign of heart disease and wonders if he should have an angiogram.

Did I mention Harry is 92?

When I graduated from medical school and started my residency over 40 years ago, there were no 90-year-olds in hospitals or cardiology clinics. The few around got their pictures in the newspaper and were tightly ensconced in clean sheets and blankets at local "nursing homes." They were, in effect, beyond any consideration of active treatment.

Since then, there has been a remarkable transformation. According to Statistics Canada, over 770,000 people over the age of 85 were living in our country in 2016. This figure had increased by 19.4 percent since 2011, which is four times the growth rate for the overall Canadian population. It's projected that by 2051, the number will exceed 2.7 million, representing 5.7 percent of the population.[4]

This is all a testament to our increasing life expectancy arising from improvements in medical management of virtually all conditions, as well as from widespread application of preventive measures and early disease detection. As my new friend Harry illustrates, his cohort is also living much more active lives and, not unreasonably, expects diagnosis and active treatment when it's required and feasible. That, of course, comes with a cost. Few are as fortunate as Harry. Most, in fact, have multiple and complex medical issues that require ongoing attention, plus long lists of medications that require regular review and renewal. The great burden of that work falls not to cardiologists and other specialists, but to family doctors.

---

[4] Statistics Canada. (2017). *2016 Census of Population: Age and sex release*. Retrieved from https://www12.statcan.gc.ca/census-recensement/2016/as-sa/98-200-x/2016004/98-200-x2016004-eng.cfm

Harry, as it turned out, had a narrowing of one of his heart valves. Over the next few months, it progressed, and his symptoms worsened. He underwent a number of diagnostic tests and eventually came to have a transcutaneous (through the skin) replacement of his valve using a guided catheter (transcuteanous aortic valve implantation, or TAVI). He tolerated all this well and is now back to enjoying his golf and travel. Twenty years ago, this would not have been possible and this still remains beyond the realm of possibility in many parts of the world. But it is possible here in North America, and, at considerable expense, physician intervention and hospital time we were successful in keeping Harry active and back on the golf course. He's very grateful, and everyone involved in his care is happy to see him doing well.

Harry is a single but useful illustration of what's required to maintain the commitment to universal health care in Canada. That burden falls to all health care providers, but certainly to physicians, and particularly to those providing primary care. Put simply, the aging and growth of our population and the rising number of therapeutic options available for previously untreatable conditions has drastically increased the burden of work expected of the medical profession, which has simply not grown in parallel.

Beyond the simple burden of increased workload, physicians are subject to continuing professional obligations. This became clearer to me after a recent conversation with a friend who had the temerity to point out (as only a true friend can) that doctors can become somewhat self-absorbed and consumed with their own "specialness." It was also his observation that they develop a certain blindness to issues of public concern or, at the very least, impose their own interpretation on such issues. During a time when the profession and government are engaged in rather intense dialogue on many public concerns, it's certainly not difficult to find examples.

At about the same time, another friend (a physician in this case), dropped an article on my desk with the notation, "I thought of you when I read this." The article was entitled "Ministerial Ethics: A Matter of Character, Conduct or Code?" and was written by Joe E. Trull, Associate Professor of Christian Ethics at the New Orleans Baptist Theological Seminary. Being unfamiliar with both Mr. Trull and the literature on ministerial ethics, I was quite intrigued by my friend's perceived connection between me and the paper's topic. The article points out that the issues being engaged by clergy as they undertake their professional roles are remarkably similar to those facing the medical profession and, by extension, to many groups that we might characterize as "professions."

How does this play out in today's world? Let's consider the following incident:

Three medical students find their way to a local pub not far from the school campus. The pub is crowded and loud. They've come directly from their classes, and so are wearing white jackets and identification badges. Over a few rounds of beers and nachos, they share their recent experiences and their perspectives on the relative attributes and shortcomings of their instructors, punctuated by animated impressions and raucous bouts of laughter. They've enjoyed the evening immensely and returned home grateful for the opportunity to "let off steam" with sympathetic colleagues.

The next day, they're called to the office of the dean of the medical school. Their conversation has been overheard by a number of town folk who easily recognized them as medical students. One of them recognizes a critically ill patient they had been discussing as a relative admitted to the hospital. To make matters worse, that person recorded parts of the conversation, and the dean has been sent the recordings by the local television station that is planning to air them on the evening news. The dean is being asked to comment.

The dean informs the students that they have breached the professionalism and confidentiality standards of the school. The matter will be reviewed by a designated panel and a number of sanctions will be considered, including expulsion from the medical program.

In the long formal review that follows, it's found that even though the students never mentioned any patient's name, they have, indeed, shared information that could readily be identified through inference and, therefore, should have been kept confidential. They are also accused of behavior that reflected badly on the school and profession.

Is this fair? Should three young people be held to a "higher standard" of conduct simply because they've chosen a particular profession? What does it even mean to be a member of a "profession"?

Historically, the term "profession" was initially applied to clergy, medicine and law, groups entrusted respectively with the spiritual welfare, physical health, and personal rights of all citizens. Many other groups have emerged with responsibility for other areas of social concern, such as nursing, engineering, architecture, pharmacy, and dentistry, to name a few. All are similarly described as "professions," a term that has come to identify groups of individuals whose role in society is primarily to provide a needed service or role, with a degree of commitment to that cause which goes beyond their personal, individual interests. People who engage in such roles are said to be "professionals," and the concept of "professionalism" is ingrained in the values and training of such groups. It can also be said that any person who engages in an occupation in a manner that puts the interest of those served above personal interests is practicing in a "professional" manner. The person who comes in the middle of a cold winter night to fix your furnace or re-establish your power supply can be said to be doing so, at least in part, because of a recognition of your critical need, and is therefore providing you a "professional" service.

There are several practical features that characterize a profession.

Professions are understood to possess certain knowledge and skills. A profession and its members are acknowledged to be the experts within that domain. They have authority over what is accepted dogma and practice and what is not.

Professions either fully control or strongly influence educational processes that recruit and educate individuals who wish to join that profession—these same recruitment and educational processes keep out others seeking to join the profession.

These educational processes always entail some component of practical training within the practice setting—a derivation of the traditional apprenticeship.

Professions have societies or organizations that define and maintain standards of practice, define methods by which those standards can be demonstrated, and publicly identify individuals who have achieved them. Membership in those organizations is accepted by society as evidence of competence.

There are also several more personal attributes and values that have been identified with professions. Professions are often characterized as "vocations." The term implies that those drawn to practice professions are somehow "called" to do so. It suggests that they perceive, for whatever reason, a sense of deep and personal purpose in the engagement of that work. It further implies that those engaging professions view their work as an important service to society and perceive that service as their main purpose and source of fulfillment in life. People who "profess" to serve within a particular domain commit to do so whenever and however the opportunity to serve may arise. It's significant that the very word "profession" has dual meanings: not only is it a "special occupation," but it is also an "avowal, or promise" (significantly, the word derives from the Latin *profiteri* meaning "to declare openly" and was first used in English around 1200 with the meaning "vows taken upon entering a religious order").

Professions are afforded a considerable degree of autonomy, which relates to several practical considerations. Established members of professions best understand their cognitive and skill-based "turf." They are therefore essential to teaching the "turf" to others. Their practical experience makes them best suited to define the standards of practice of the profession and to identify the personal qualities that characterize those best suited to enter and practice the profession and to characterize the qualities of those not suited to its membership.

But above these practical considerations, the autonomy arises from a societal trust that those "called" to practice a profession are motivated solely by the desire to ensure that the quality of that service is maintained for all who require it. In the words of Eliot Freidson, author of *Profession of Medicine: A Study of the Sociology of Applied Knowledge,* "the occupation sustains its special status by its persuasive profession of the extraordinary trustworthiness of its members."[5]

But this "extraordinary trustworthiness" comes with a price. There exists an understandable suite of societal expectations expressed toward any autonomous professional group.

Responsible professionals:

- Do not withhold their service from those in need.
- Do not withhold their service for the purpose of personal gain.
- Can be relied upon to provide the highest quality work and recognize when they have fallen short.
- Ensure their knowledge and skills are maintained.
- Commit to their responsibilities regardless of clock or calendar.
- Ensure continuity of their responsibilities when they themselves are no longer able to provide.
- Ensure public trust and faith in the profession.

A tall order, for sure. In the past, when doctors practiced almost exclusively as individual practitioners, these obligations could be met only through tremendous personal sacrifice.

And so, those who "profess" to be doctors in our society bear both burdens—those related to the increased workload of providing an expanding array of services to an expanding and aging population, as

---

[5] Freidson, E. (1970). *Profession of Medicine: A Study of the Sociology of Applied Knowledge.* University of Chicago Press, p. XV.

well as the behavioral and personal obligations that go with belonging to a venerable and essential profession.

At the same time, doctors themselves are changing. They are embracing a very understandable desire to protect their personal time and health. The concept of physician "wellness" has become a central consideration of most of those who practice medicine and is even finding its way into mission statements and curricula of medical schools and training programs.

This is all understandable, but the result is an inescapable tension between increasing societal demands and a desire for physicians and the physician community to protect the health and autonomy of its members.

All this is particularly relevant to the theme of this book, because family doctors who provide that "comprehensive, continuing" care to their patients are among the most vulnerable when it comes to keeping their own wellbeing secure. Their commitment to their patients is not bounded by time or the completion of a particular service. As such, they serve as the default primary caregivers for the patient when other specialists are unable to adequately address the patient's needs that extend beyond their specialized areas of practice.

At my last clinic appointment with Harry, I found he was feeling much better, and his new valve was functioning well. At the end of the appointment, as he was buttoning up his shirt, he asked:

"Doc, would you mind looking at this mole on my neck? It's been getting bigger and began bleeding the other day? Also, I've been having trouble sleeping? Anything you can suggest?"

As a cardiologist, I have the option of suggesting Harry book an appointment with his family doctor to discuss those two concerns. Everyone, including Harry, would understand that. In fact, in doing so, I would be acting responsibly, within my expected "scope of practice."

Harry's family doctor does not have that option.

CHAPTER FOUR

The Contemporary Physician

The Norman Rockwell Doctor

NORMAN ROCKWELL WAS BORN IN New York City in 1894 and never strayed far from his birthplace during his long career as a highly prolific painter and illustrator. He's best remembered for his depictions of the mid-20th-century American culture. Although hugely popular, his work is considered by many, including serious art critics, to be idealistic and overly sentimental. Among his works are several illustrations of doctors at work. The doctors of Mr. Rockwell's world were invariably male, white, middle-aged, benevolent, formally dressed, and dealing with patients who didn't seem particularly ill.

Although certainly idealized and far from realistic, Mr. Rockwell's image of the iconic physician was consistent with other portrayals appearing in popular culture at the time. Ben Casey, Dr. Kildare, and even Dr. "Bones" McCoy of *Star Trek* fame all kept to the script of the all-paternal, all-knowing, always-available physician. With time, fictional doctors have become more diverse in gender and culture, more obviously stressed and emotional, but the image of complete, unchallenged knowledge and self-sacrificing dedication has persisted.

And so, for that generation of Canadians now referred to as "baby boomers" who form a huge and impactful force in our society, an image was fermented of the ideal physician.

- Doctors were assumed to have complete knowledge of any medical issue that might arise.
- Every individual and every family in a community had "their doctor" with whom they were bonded, literally from "cradle to grave."
- They were *always* available. There were no "office hours." They could always be reached.
- Doctors worked alone, in private and separate practices. They must have had some way of sharing responsibilities, because on the rare occasion that need arose while your doctor was away, one of his colleagues would somehow magically appear. It wasn't clear how that came about.
- They handled everything medical, from deliveries to minor ailments, to fractures, to surgeries to emergencies, through to end-of-life care and bereavement counseling to families.
- They made decisions about what could or could not be done about any medical issue.
- They had authority. Their decisions seemed beyond questioning. This is not so much that they were unwilling to discuss their decisions, but rather that the opportunity never arose because, for most patients, to do so was not something they would consider.
- They knew their patients medically and personally. They were often called upon to provide personal references and, I've no doubt, to provide personal guidance.

- They were pillars of the community. Every community council, every school board, every library committee, and every fundraising effort, included at least one doctor. And they were listened to, not because they necessarily had authoritative knowledge of the subject under discussion, but because they could be relied upon to understand and express in an unbiased way the best interests of the community.
- It was assumed, based on their training and behavior, that they were motivated by a greater purpose than simply earning a livelihood and so could be trusted to put the welfare of their patients and community above all other interests.

But, as we all know, things have metamorphosed from this idyllic state. To illustrate, let's meet Maria, who's waiting to see her new doctor.

Maria's Story

Maria had been waiting almost four weeks for this appointment. She's quite nervous about it. She's only met her new doctor once before and that was for something called an "intake interview." For that, she was required to fill out many forms in advance that seemed to explore all aspects of her medical and personal history. Since Maria is now 84, there was a lot to remember, and many parts had to be left blank or simply filled in with a "not sure." She found her new doctor to be courteous, efficient and, it seemed to Maria, very young. Maria guessed the doctor to be about the same age as her granddaughter. At the first interview, they reviewed the items Maria had been able to complete in the "intake inventory."

Her high blood pressure and medications she was taking for it.

The breast cancer she had 15 years ago and how it had been treated with surgery and radiation (Maria couldn't remember how many treatments she had undergone).

Her three pregnancies and how difficult the last one had been, with a need for hospitalization before delivery.

How difficult it had been for her when her husband, Dave, died 5 years ago. Her previous doctor had seen her several times and prescribed a medication "for her nerves." Maria couldn't remember the name of the medication.

Her history of flu shots and shingles vaccine and the reaction she had after one of them, which caused a painful, swollen arm and peeling skin. She remembers very clearly how concerned Dave had become, finally taking her to the emergency department late one night. She couldn't remember exactly when or which vaccination it had been, but there must be a record somewhere.

It seemed to Maria they had discussed each of these items as someone might review a grocery list, without particular emphasis or elaboration at any point. As they spoke, the doctor was typing, eyes focused on the computer screen positioned on her desk in such a way that she could shift her gaze easily from the screen to Maria. Maria felt like the third party in the room, the more important interaction being between the doctor and the computer. The cadence and clicking of the keyboard signaled when attention turned to her, when it was her turn to talk. Each "item" they reviewed re-awakened memories and feelings that were still raw and poignant even after so many years, but none of that seemed at all relevant to the purpose of the "intake interview."

She couldn't help comparing the new doctor to her old doctor who had looked after her, Dave, and the children since they'd moved to this community many years ago. Her former family doctor was a constant, reliable presence in the backdrop of their lives, emerging when the need arose, whether it was in the office, delivery room, or hospital. The office encounters were "visits," with no need to review and re-review past events, and certainly no typing or computer screens interfered back then. Maria wasn't sure how she was going to manage when he retired last year but was reassured when he told her he was transferring his practice to a new doctor who was very well qualified. Maria knew that many of her friends were not so fortunate and were left without new doctors when theirs had stopped practicing altogether.

And so, she now found herself in the same waiting room she'd had known for so many years, but hardly recognizable with the redesign and refurbishing. It was much brighter. The big and clunky chairs had been replaced with efficient modular seating with the result that the room could now hold many more people than it had previously. The old wooden desk where the receptionist sat and greeted people by name as they came in was replaced with a glass screen that separated the staff, and their computer screens, from the waiting area. People spoke through an opening in the glass and Maria was required, each time, to produce her health card and confirm the address of the home she'd been living in for several decades. There were numerous signs and notices on the walls that spoke to office procedures, regulations, schedules of after-hours clinics and that reminded people to wash their hands and wear a mask if they felt unwell.

As Maria waited, she felt the need to be more efficient and precise with the new doctor than she'd been last time and so she went over in her mind the things that were concerning her.

She had a dark spot on her upper chest that she'd had thought was a mole, but it seemed to be getting larger and, a couple of times, began bleeding when she inadvertently scratched it. Could it be a skin cancer? Her friend Brenda had gone to her doctor with a smaller spot and was sent to a surgeon to have it removed.

She'd not been sleeping well. She was going to bed at the usual time but waking up at about one or two in the morning and not able to get to back to sleep. She had gotten into the habit of watching old movies at night and then felt exhausted by noon the next day. That couldn't be normal, could it? It seemed to start when she found some water seepage in the basement of the house and her son told her she'd need to get a contractor to look at it. Dave had always taken care of such things.

She'd been having headaches, too, which is a new experience for her. In fact, she'd always been able to boast that she didn't even know what a headache was. She certainly did now. Most days, there was a pounding behind her eyes that seemed to extend to the back of her head. She was using Tylenol regularly, but it wasn't helping much. She'd mentioned it to her daughter, who insisted she make this appointment.

And so here she was, with her three problems well rehearsed in her mind, prepared to review them efficiently during the appointment, and not take up too much of her doctor's time.

And then she saw the sign. It was over the opening in the glass barrier, and she'd missed it as she was producing her health card for the receptionist. But there it was:

"One problem per visit please."

One problem? Which one? How was she to decide? Maybe the one she'd had the longest? Her daughter would be very upset if she didn't report that she'd mentioned the headaches. Maria became confused and panicky. As her name was called to see the doctor, she was close to tears.

Maria's Doctor

Maria's new doctor is Tamara. She's 30 years old and she's recently taken over her first independent medical practice as a fully qualified family physician.

Tamara grew up in an affluent neighborhood of a large city. Her father is a retired lawyer. Her mother is a retired high school principal, now engaged in several volunteer activities, including the board of directors of a local hospital. Sarah has one younger sister, who is an investment banker.

Tamara attended private elementary and high schools. During her elementary school years, she took piano lessons and was active in both figure skating and horseback riding. In high school, she excelled academically and participated in several extracurricular activities. She was an accomplished athlete, breaking two school track and field records, and was a member of the varsity team that won a provincial championship.

At some point in high school, she began to consider applying to medical school. She's not exactly sure how or when it started but, as she began to talk about becoming a doctor, everyone seemed to feel it was a perfect fit for her. Her parents, guidance counselors, and friends were uniformly supportive and encouraging, convinced that it was a perfect career for a young woman with so much natural ability and academic drive. Medical school admission, everyone realized, was very difficult to achieve, but Sarah, everyone agreed, had the intelligence and scholastic tenacity to achieve any goal she set her mind to. And so, she went about researching the medical school admission process, and what she would have to do to be successful.

She learned that she would be able to apply to medical school only after obtaining a university degree and that she would have to get very good marks in her university courses, have a record of experiences that would impress an admissions committee, and do very well in an examination called the Medical College Admission Test, or MCAT. And so, she and her parents went about ensuring all was in place for her to ensure a successful application.

After carefully reviewing universities and published rankings, they chose one that was considered academically prestigious and had a highly regarded medical school. She chose an academic program and courses that would both demonstrate an interest in medical science and allow her the opportunity to achieve very high marks that they felt would be needed. She sought out community and volunteer opportunities that would allow her to learn more about health care and medicine, while demonstrating her commitment to community service, even though it meant giving up her athletics and horseback riding. She learned about the admission test she'd be required to take and prepared for it by purchasing manuals and taking courses that were provided to prepare applicants for success in the examination. All this was very expensive and didn't allow any time for part-time jobs but, fortunately for Tamara, her parents were well off financially and more than happy to support her goals.

Tamara was successful in getting accepted into medical school, to her delight and the delight of her parents, family, and friends. All agreed this was as it should be, nor was it surprising to anyone in her social circle. She would become a great doctor.

In medical school, she continued to fare well academically, particularly in the basic and clinical science courses in the first and second years. She had no difficulty learning the concepts, remembering the key information and organizing the material in ways that allow her to easily pass the numerous examinations.

She had more difficulty when she began to encounter and examine patients. She found she wasn't comfortable encountering people she didn't already know, particularly older people or anyone who wasn't able to answer her questions clearly. She found that frustrating. She also had difficulty with clinical problems that didn't have a clear right or wrong answer. The concept that the best approach to a patient problem might differ for different patients depending on their circumstances and "preferences" was perplexing to her. Surely, there must be a single right answer? Isn't that what a "science" is about? For the first time, she began to question whether this was, in fact, the right career for her. She decided to discuss her concerns with a counselor, who reassured her that these reactions were common and even natural in students these days and should improve as her training progresses. Even if they didn't, the counselor went on to say, there are many ways to practice medicine in which those troubling patient encounters could be minimized.

Tamara also learned about the importance of something called work–life balance. It was very important, she learned, to ensure that the demands of medical school and a medical career did not overwhelm and consume all her energy and interests. She was cautioned to be vigilant in protecting her personal time and ensuring her energy and personal interests were not consumed by her career. The two, she came to believe, are playing a tug-of-war, in which she is the rope. The consequences of losing the struggle, she learned, are dire and include a condition called burnout.

All this came to a head when she had to decide what medical specialty to pursue after medical school. Her natural inclination was to pursue a specialty that is highly procedural in order to minimize new patient encounters and ongoing contacts. But she was also attracted to programs with shorter training times and more career flexibility.

And something else has happened along the way. She met Marcus. Marcus is a classmate she began seeing socially, and the two developed a special relationship. With time, they became committed to each other romantically and planned to remain together through their training and beyond. Marcus decided to pursue residency in vascular surgery. Based on the availability of training spots and length of that residency, it became clear to both of them that their ability to remain together and ability to perhaps have children (which was important to Marcus) would be much improved if Tamara took on a shorter training program with fewer "on call" requirements. And so, Tamara went into a family medicine training program. Even though she took a year off to have a child, she completed the program while Marcus was in his residency.

As she completed her residency, a career opportunity came to their attention in the same community in which they were training.

During her residency, Tamara had gotten to know an older family physician who was about to retire and was seeking a new graduate to take over his practice. His practice was about to become part of a newly formed "Family Health Team," which meant it would combine several other family practices to develop a common clinic, shared support staff, and access to a number of allied health professionals (including a physician assistant, physiotherapist, nutritionist, and pharmacist) to deliver care to a large population of "enrolled" patients. Tamara saw this as an excellent opportunity to start practice in a way she could manifest control over how patients are scheduled and seen and be able to work with and share responsibilities with other doctors. She eagerly participated in the redesign of the workspace to make it more efficient, and she led the effort to convert all medical records to an electronic, computer-based system with no further need for paper-based records.

The "one-problem-per-visit" policy, she felt, would perfectly fit the dual need to maintain office efficiency and safeguard the work–life balance she had learned to cherish. It will ensure smooth and efficient patient flow and optimize the use of shared, limited resources, she felt, while also shielding her and other physicians from undue stress and long hours. As Maria is led into her office, Tamara is eager to hear about and engage in whatever single problem her patient chooses to present her with, fingers poised at her keyboard.

Older Patients, Younger Doctors: Demographics of the Doctor–Patient Relationship

This little drama between Maria and her new doctor, Tamara, illustrates many of the changes that have occurred in both patients and doctors over the past few decades. Let's examine some of those changes.

In 1960, the average life expectancy of the 18 million Canadians was about 71 years, and about 3.8 percent of them were over the age of 65. In 2015, 38 million Canadians are living an average of 82 years, and the percentage over the age of 65 has increased to almost 17 percent, with projections for it to reach 25 percent by 2050. A few years ago, the number of seniors in Canada exceeded the number of children for the first time in history. What does all this mean for the doctor–patient interaction? A few decades ago, the typical doctor was usually older than their patient. That is reversing itself. Today, and even more so into the future, younger physicians will be looking after older patients—in fact, much older patients.

The percentage of women in the physician workforce has increased dramatically over the past few decades. In 1970, it was about 7 percent. According to a 2019 report by Canadian Medical Association, 43% of physicians in Canada were women and that women accounted for almost two-thirds (64%) of physicians under the age of 35.[6] The Canadian Institute for Health Information reported in 2022 that half of family physicians in Canada are female, but were younger than their male counterparts (47 vs 50 years).[7] Given that medical school enrolment is at least equally divided between men and women, those figures are sure to rise with increasing age differences in the future. Since women dominate in older age groups generally in our society, the most common doctor–patient mix in future years will be a younger female physician, matched with a much older, female patient.

---

[6] Canadian Medical Association. (n.d.). *Quick facts: Canada's physicians*. Retrieved from https://www.cma.ca/quick-facts-canadas-physicians#:~:text=Physician%20mix&text=43%25%20are%20female%3B%2057%25,school%2C%203%25%20not%20stated

[7] Canadian Institute for Health Information. (n.d.). *A profile of physicians in Canada*. Retrieved from https://www.cihi.ca/en/a-profile-of-physicians-in-canada#:~:text=Text%20version%20of%20infographic&text=Overall%2C%20the%20average%20age%20of,previous%20year%20to%20%2430.8%20billion

All this means that whereas the typical physician of the 1960s was a male much older than his patient, the typical physician of the mid-21st century will be a woman providing care to a much older patient, usually another woman. This fundamental demographic reversal must fundamentally change the very nature of the relationship. It will also change many assumptions about the very purpose of the relationship. The issues of end-of-life care and "quality versus quantity" of life, for example, are becoming much more relevant and even essential elements of the discussion today and tomorrow than they were in years past.

At the same time, there's much more medical work for a family doctor to do.

Thanks to great advances in medical science and improved living conditions, people are now living longer and better. Conditions for which there were few or no treatments many years ago, such as diabetes, cardiac disease, kidney disease, and cancer, are now very treatable, but those treatments can be complex and lifelong. As a result of the combined effects of more people, longer lives, and more treatments required, there's a consequent dramatic increase in the burden of work falling to the entire medical community, much of which is carried out by family physicians.

In addition, there's a greatly heightened awareness of the importance of preventing many diseases, particular cardiac disease, cancer, and various infectious illness, through vaccination. Although it can rightfully be argued that all specialists should be promoting prevention in their practices, that burden falls most directly on family medicine and primary care.

The net effect is that there is more medical care required for more people.

Doctors are no longer willing, nor should they be reasonably expected, to devote all their time and energy to their practice. They want to provide good care *and* preserve their personal time, interests, and relationships. To do so, they seek to improve efficiency through the use of technology and by establishing firm boundaries between their personal and professional lives. To make matters worse, the number of doctors in Canada has grown over the years, but proportionately much less than the population growth. Currently, the ratio of doctors to population in Canada (242 per 100,000) ranks 22nd among countries, and is less than half that of many.[8]

The net result of these two parallel developments is that society's needs are increasing, while the capacity of the medical profession to provide those needs is not growing in tandem.

Something has to give, and the consequences are playing out in countless interactions such as that between Maria and Tamara. That mismatch also contributes, to a large extent, to the increasing number of patients unable to access a family physician.

All this leads to only a couple of potential approaches proposed by policy makers. One is to simply produce more doctors, hoping to match the need through increased supply. We are essentially engaging in this strategy when decisions are made to increase the number of medical schools or positions within each school. However, the benefit to the supply of the sort of family doctors that are required will be very limited since, as we've seen, only a small proportion of students (probably less than 20 percent) engaged in our current programs ultimately choose to become family physicians devoted to that continuing, community-based practice described throughout this book as being fundamental to holistic patient care. Consequently, increasing the numbers entering the current training process will have limited impact. It will also have the effect of increasing the numbers within other specialties, regardless of societal need. Expansion, to be effective, must be done in the context of

---

[8] The Global Economy. (n.d.). *Doctors per 1,000 people by country*. Retrieved from https://www.theglobaleconomy.com/rankings/doctors_per_1000_people/

a fundamental reconsideration of *who* is admitted, to what *purpose* they are admitted, and *how* they are trained.

The other common approach is to increase the efficiency of family physicians in practice, thus allowing them to take care of more patients and doing so in a way that meets their personal needs and expectations. As our previous accounts have suggested, there are many opportunities to achieve this, while improving patient access and satisfaction, by re-thinking the underlying model of care delivery in which family doctors are involved. As Aristotle might say, a systematic examination demands a reimagining of the parameters.

More on both of these approaches in later chapters when we explore potential solutions. For now, let's look further into the practice environment and how the skills required of today's doctors have changed since the Norman Rockwell era of doctoring.

CHAPTER FIVE

Out of One, Many

AS RECENTLY AS 60 YEARS ago, a typical Canadian family could get along quite nicely with one income, one car, one television, one telephone, and one doctor. Their expectation was that their doctor would be always available, for all members of the family young and old, and would address any medical issue that might befall them.

Clearly, much has changed. Advances in medical care have been staggeringly successful in reducing the burden of disease and allowing us to live longer and enjoy more active lives. With those changes, the medical profession has evolved and diversified. No longer can a single doctor provide all aspects of care that a patient might require over the course of their life. No longer is medicine symbolized by a homogeneous type of doctor or as an independent undertaking. The term "medical doctor" now applies to well over a hundred different interdependent specialties and areas of interest.

Jamie's Story

Jamie is a 24-year-old college student who has always been in good health. She shares an apartment with two other young women and, one evening, admits to them over dinner that she's been feeling "off" all day. One of her roommates, who's a nursing student, asks what she means by this. Jamie has difficulty describing it more clearly but indicates that she's been a little more short of breath and wasn't able to finish her usual jog that afternoon. She's also been having some jabbing pains in her chest when she breathes. She thinks it might just be because she's been up late studying for mid-terms and has become overtired. The next morning, she's no better. In fact, she's grown a little worse. At her roommate's insistence and with her help, she decides to see the doctor at Student Health.

The doctor at the college's Student Health office is a local family physician who works at the college one day a week. He's not met Jamie previously but asks some questions about her recent and past health, what medications she's taking, and the level of stress in her life. He also takes her blood pressure and listens to her heart and lungs with his stethoscope. He's not sure what's going on but is concerned that she doesn't look well and arranges for her to have a chest X-ray and "breathing tests." He gives Jamie requisitions for both and sends her to the nearby university hospital to have both tests carried out.

Later that afternoon, a radiologist at the hospital reviews Jamie's X-ray and calls the family physician at the college. He's alarmed about the appearance and is worried that Jamie might have a blood clot in her lungs (a pulmonary embolism). The college doctor then contacts Jamie to ask how she's feeling. Jamie admits that she's been getting worse over the course of the day, and the doctor notices that she seems a little short of breath on the phone. Based on that, and the X-ray findings, he advises Jamie to go to the emergency room (ER) of the university hospital and calls the doctor on duty at that time to let her know that Jamie is coming and about his concerns.

The emergency physician sees Jamie shortly after she arrives, examines her again, and explains to her that they're concerned about the pulmonary embolism, which could certainly account for her symptoms, and that she should be treated urgently to avoid further problems. She orders blood work and arranges for Jamie to have an urgent CT scan. Jamie is taken by stretcher to the radiology department and, after getting an injection of material to visualize her pulmonary vessels, undergoes the imaging scan. Just as the scan is complete, she begins to feel severe pains in her chest and experiences much more shortness of breath. She is rushed back to the emergency department where, over the course of the next hour, a lung specialist (respirologist) and intensive care specialist are consulted. She is started on a series of treatments that include intravenous medications intended to dissolve the clot. But because Jamie's breathing has not improved with an oxygen mask and her blood pressure is dropping, she is sedated and has a tube passed into her airway to support her ventilation. In the meantime, another radiologist has read the CT scan and confirmed that Jamie has a "massive" pulmonary embolism entirely blocking blood flow to one of her lungs. It's so large, in fact, that any further embolism might be fatal.

Meanwhile, Jamie had an urgent echocardiogram (cardiac ultrasound) carried out in the ER. A cardiologist has reviewed it and called the ER physician to say it shows changes to the size and function of the right side of Jamie's heart, which is likely related to a large pulmonary embolism. Based on all this, the ER physician and intensivist (intensive care medicine specialist) jointly make the decision to ask the interventional radiologist on duty that day to insert a device into one of Jamie's blood vessels (the inferior vena cava, the largest vein in the body) to block any further clots from getting to her lungs. Jamie then spends the next week in the intensive care unit (ICU) where she gradually recovers. Over that time, she's cared for by an intensivist. In addition, a cardiologist (heart specialist) and hematologist (blood specialist) are consulted who provide further advice about her care. She makes a good recovery and is transferred out of ICU to a medical ward, where she is under the care of a general internist. Before going home, she sees a medical geneticist to determine if she may have an inherited condition that predisposes her to blood clots. She is also seen by a rehabilitation medicine specialist for advice about increasing activity and is transferred to the local rehabilitation hospital for a few days to recover fully before returning home. After discharge, she will need to remain on many medications and be followed by both her family physician and hematologist. She'll also need to be seen by another interventional radiologist to have the filter removed.

Jamie's story is a medical success story. She had a very serious, life-threatening illness, but received excellent care and had an excellent outcome. Now, let's tally up the various doctors that were involved in Jamie's treatment:

1. Family physician at student health
2. Radiologist who interpreted the initial x-ray
3. ER physician
4. Second radiologist who interpreted the CT scan
5. Respirologist who was called to see her in the ER
6. Intensive care specialist who saw her in the ER
7. Cardiologist who interpreted her echocardiogram
8. Interventional radiologist who implanted the filter
9. Attending intensivist in the ICU
10. Hematologist who consulted in the ICU
11. Medical geneticist
12. General internist attending on the medical ward
13. Rehabilitation specialist

In the course of that illness, she was treated by no fewer than thirteen different doctors, representing eleven different discrete medical specialties. She found them all to be very courteous and efficient but, by the time she gets home, she's unable to recall the name of even one. In fact, the only doctor she can recall with any clarity is the family physician at student health who initially referred her to the hospital.

The Evolution of Specialization

At one point, doctors all underwent the same medical education, and all practiced in very similar ways, with the same scope of activity and responsibilities. To illustrate how much the medical landscape has evolved, it might be useful to consider a "Tale of Three Classes" who have graduated from the Queen's University School of Medicine in Kingston, Ontario.

This photograph provided by the Queen's University Archives illustrates one of the earliest graduating classes, circa 1865. Students of that era received a common three to four years of instruction and clinical training, after which they become fully qualified practitioners. Their scope of practice throughout their careers was virtually identical, determined only by the needs of the communities they served.

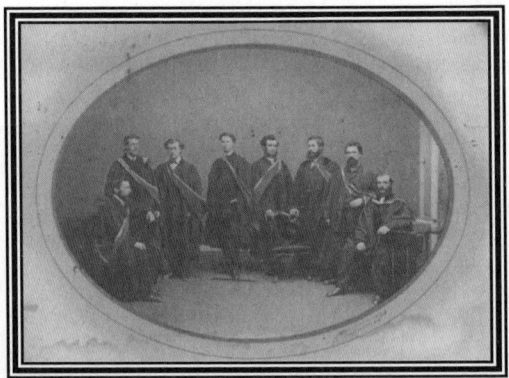

Class of 1865, School of Medicine, Queen's University

Let's move forward about a hundred years. The second photo was taken at the 25th reunion of my class, Meds '81. My classmates and I also undertook a common four-year curriculum. With one further year of training, in virtually any "internship," we were all deemed fully qualified as "general practitioners." About half the class remained in general practice, eventually becoming qualified by the College of Family Physicians when that body and its qualifying examinations came into being. The remainder went on to additional training in one of the limited number of specialty programs and certification examinations offered by the Royal College of Physicians and Surgeons. Importantly, I doubt any of my contemporaries regretted their general training, and even those eventually engaged in very specialized disciplines would say that their clinical proficiency and effectiveness were enhanced by that background.

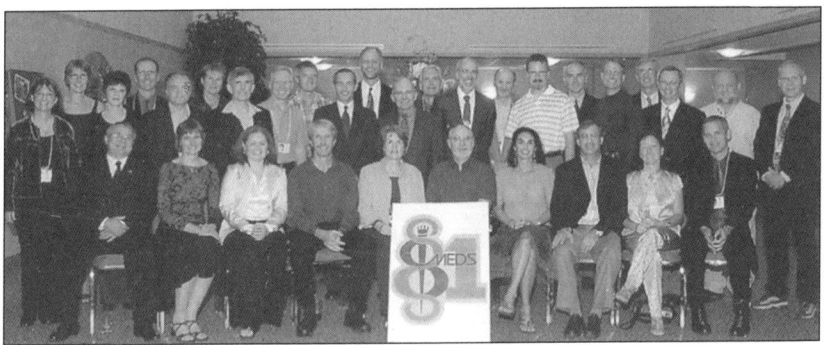

25th Reunion of Class of 1981, School of Medicine, Queen's University

Contrast all this to the graduates of Meds 2009. About a quarter of these students undertook training in family medicine. They completed the two- or three-year training program and then passed the qualifying examination to achieve certification with the College of Family Physicians.

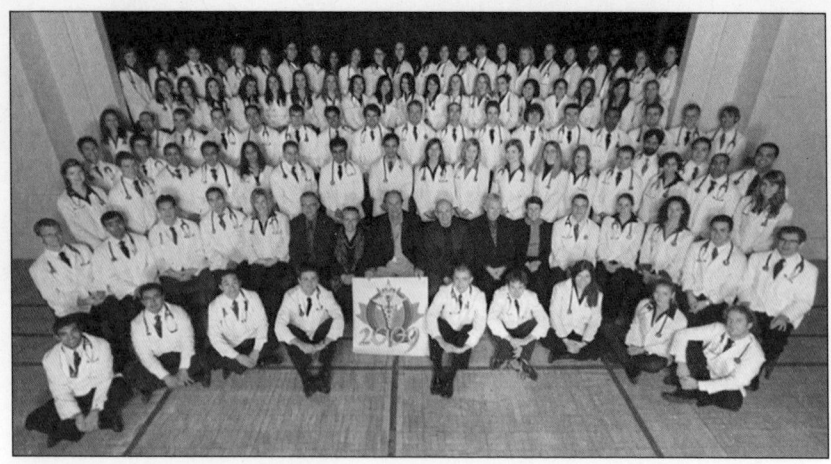

Class of 2009, School of Medicine, Queen's University

The remainder chose, at graduation, to enter one of the nearly thirty distinct training programs offered by the Royal College of Physicians and Surgeons of Canada. These include:

- Anesthesiology
- Anatomical pathology
- Cardiac surgery
- Dermatology
- Diagnostic radiology
- Emergency medicine
- General pathology
- General surgery
- Hematological pathology
- Internal medicine
- Laboratory medicine
- Medical genetics
- Medical microbiology
- Neurology
- Neurology—pediatric

- Neuropathology
- Neurosurgery
- Nuclear medicine
- Obstetrics and gynecology
- Ophthalmology
- Orthopedics
- Otolaryngology
- Pediatrics
- Physical medicine and rehabilitation
- Plastic surgery
- Public health and preventive medicine
- Psychiatry
- Radiation oncology
- Urology
- Vascular surgery

In addition, many of these "primary-entry" disciplines further differentiate themselves into various other specialties and subspecialties. Trainees in internal medicine, for example, can elect to finish their training after four years and become general internists, or engage further training after two or three years in any of the following:

- Allergy
- Cardiology
- Endocrinology
- Gastroenterology
- Hematology
- Infectious disease
- Nephrology
- Oncology
- Respirology
- Rheumatology

The world of medicine is becoming even more complex as knowledge, technologies and new areas of care emerge. My own specialty of cardiology is a particularly illustrative example. When I initially qualified, all cardiologists basically did the same job, saw the same patient population, and provided the same spectrum of services. Today, interventional cardiology, electrophysiology, imaging and heart failure have all evolved as distinct areas of sub-sub-specialization, all with emerging training requirements that the Royal College is beginning to formally recognize. Consequently, the journey through to practice readiness for someone who practices as a cardiologist with special skills in imaging might look like this:

Medical school (3-4 years)
→ **Internal medicine residency (3 years)**
→ **Cardiology residency (3 years)**
→ **Imaging fellowship (1-2 years)**

All this can take up to 12 years after entering medical school, or 16 years after starting university, since most people complete an undergraduate degree before entering medical school. If they choose to be involved in research, additional years may be involved to obtain a master's or PhD.

Importantly, the training becomes increasingly specific and more closely related to the ultimate practice as it progresses. Conversely, early education becomes less relevant as training progresses. This process has developed not intentionally, but rather because as more specific disciplines and medical applications have evolved, they have grown from and therefore been grafted onto existing specialty training programs, which always require a medical degree as a key admission criterion.

The student who goes on to practice family medicine is much more likely to utilize and benefit from what was learned in medical school than one who undertakes one of the Royal College specialties. The problem, of course, is that neither of these types of students, in their pre-medicine days, knows what they wish to do when they enter medical school. In fact, much of their medical school experience is taken up with making that important selection of a career.

College student Jamie's story is not an uncommon account and illustrates the reality of modern, specialty-based medical care. Specialization represents perhaps the greatest change in the practice of medicine over the past half century. It is a function of the vast expansion of medical knowledge and has allowed the medical profession to master and provide all the new and emerging therapies effectively. It also profoundly affects the relationship between doctors and patients. Specialization essentially defines two types of physicians, the specialist and the generalist. For specialists, patient engagement begins and ends with a particular issue that falls within their area of interest and expertise. Traditional physicians, or modern-day generalists, engage the patient and whatever issue or issues may arise. The generalist is more focused on diagnosis and prevention of illness, and the specialist is more focused on reversing or minimizing the impact of illness. The specialist's unspoken contract with the patient is limited by the resolution of the specialist-defined medical issue they have been engaged to deal with. The generalist's engagement with the patient is open-ended and continuing, taken up as need arises or opportunities for prevention present themselves.

How Medical Specialties Differ

Medical specialties differ in a number of other important ways. These differences define the specialties and are the major determinant used by students in deciding which specialty to engage.

Engagement of patients with acute illness

Patients encounter doctors for one of two reasons—because an acute illness causes them to seek help or because another doctor referred them. In today's world, it is the minority of specialties, and the minority of doctors, who see patients acutely, or at the start of their illness. Examples would include family medicine, pediatrics, emergency medicine and, to some extent, intensive care. Other specialties and most doctors largely engage patients who have been previously assessed and have undergone some sort of preliminary diagnostic process and even stabilization of the clinical condition.

This has led to the development of a formalized consultancy of physicians. Consulting physicians review patients at the request of a physician who has engaged the patient initially and wishes further assistance with specific aspects of care. Consultants are seen as physicians with more expertise or specific knowledge or skill relevant to that patient's requirements. The consultant's role is therefore fundamentally very different. The consultant does not engage the patient in a holistic, comprehensive manner, but with the intention of addressing a specific need. The understanding is that the consultant's involvement is limited to the specific issue and therefore time limited. There is no obligation to engage the broader needs of the patient (such as underlying mental health concerns previously undetected), but rather to engage the patient, narrowly, focused on the particular issue for which they have been consulted.

Consultancy is highly valuable and is a standard component of modern medical care. However, it is a fundamentally different engagement. The physician consultant's professional challenge is to maintain the primacy of the patient while directing their attention to a particular clinical issue.

Continuing versus episodic care

A number of specialties engage patients in a continuing relationship. The goals of the relationship are to promote ongoing health and prevent disease as well as providing treatment of acute illness. Family physicians, pediatricians and, in some contexts, general internists engage patients on a continuing basis with the goal of maintaining health and addressing acute illnesses that may arise. Continuing relationships can also develop in the context of chronic conditions that require ongoing care, such as rheumatologic or chronic renal disease.

Most other specialties of medicine engage patient care in the context of a particular disease. The understanding is that the physician brings specific expertise that they will apply and, once the condition is resolved or it is clear that the particular treatment is no longer needed, they disengage. The role is therefore defined by the condition and not by the patients themselves.

Service or procedurally specific care
There are numerous conditions for which patients require particular procedures or interventions. A large number of patient–physician encounters are therefore now structured around the application of a particular procedure. The patient engages the physician in order to access a particular treatment. All parties involved—the service providing physician, referring physician, and patient—implicitly accept this understanding.

The relationship is therefore something of a contract for the provision of that care. It is understood by all to be limited to the application of the particular service. A patient engages an anesthesiologist, for example, because they require support through a procedure. Once that procedure is complete and the patient has fully recovered, the relationship ends.

Patient populations
Specialties differ with respect to the patient populations they serve. Pediatrics and gerontology are obvious examples. However, there are many other specialties whose activity is particular to very specific patient populations. Cardiologists, for example, largely treat

older patients. In fact, an entirely separate specialty has developed to deal with young people with cardiac illness - pediatric cardiology. Certain infectious conditions are more endemic in poorer, younger socioeconomic groups; for example, there may be elevated rates of rheumatic fever, skin infections, meningitis, and respiratory infections linked to overcrowded housing conditions and lack of access to health care. This differential impact will influence the patient population that a particular specialty may be dealing with.

Practice settings

Specialties differ with respect to practice location. Medicine can be practiced in offices, emergency departments, critical care units, operating rooms, and even in very public settings. Individual will differ remarkably in their degree of comfort in these particular environments. The operating room, for example, is obviously essential to the provision of surgical care. Individuals who undertake surgery must be comfortable with the particular procedures, pace, and intimacy of the operating room. Emergency departments are often crowded, busy, and stressful environments. Individuals will vary dramatically in their natural comfort with these settings and their degree of comfort can only be assessed after personal experience.

Shiftwork

Virtually all medical specialties require some degree of "on-call" work. (Being "on call" in medicine refers to a physician or health care provider being available and responsible for responding to patient care needs during designated time periods, typically outside of regular working hours.) In addition, some specialties must provide service round-the-clock and therefore require practitioners to engage irregular work schedules. The burden of work on call and the impact of shiftwork varies dramatically not only among specialties but among particular disciplines within specialties. Individuals vary considerably in their natural ability to work effectively under these conditions. The impact of on-call and shiftwork also changes considerably as physicians age and take on other roles in their careers and lives. In addition, physicians and those engaging medical practice early in their careers are increasingly aware of the impact of the grueling work hours on their effectiveness and on their personal lives. Learners are certainly considering these factors as they select career options in medicine.

Geographic locations
More specialized areas of practice are most usefully applied in large population areas. On the other hand, primary care practices and general practices in fields such as internal medicine and surgery, are needed in smaller communities. The specialties therefore differ with respect to the locations potentially available to practitioners.

Income
Finally, it must be recognized that the specialties vary considerably in terms of the income available to practitioners. In North America, physicians are generally compensated based on the number and types of encounters they provide, and procedural care is highly valued in most care models. This "fee-for-service" model of physician compensation has evolved historically, and it has resulted in disproportionate compensation to some specialties that have high procedural mixes, such as ophthalmology, cardiology, radiology, and many surgical disciplines. On the other hand, specialties that do not have a high procedural heterogeneity, such as family medicine, psychiatry, and pediatrics, are much less well compensated. Fundamentally, the physician who engages the patient encounter itself and clinical decision-making (arguably the most important and critical aspects of care) earn less than their colleagues who do largely procedural work.

A number of funding models have been and continue to be developed to address this, but the disparities certainly exist and are no doubt influential in career decision-making.

The Benefits of Specialization

In considering all these changes, it's important to recognize that the major driver of change is the increase in the corpus of medical knowledge, available technologies, and the vast expansion of valuable service that the profession is able to provide to patients. Our society expects that physicians will have highly specialized knowledge and training required to diagnose and manage our ever-expanding array of conditions and to provide technologically complex treatments. This is, obviously, a net benefit to everyone.

Specialization has allowed the profession to engage this dramatic service expansion. It is essentially a "divide-and-conquer" approach whereby the profession has engaged broader and vastly expanded applications. Individuals can readily focus on a particular area rather than the vast expanse of medicine and therefore develop mastery in specific domains. Patients benefit from high levels of technical expertise in services they may require. Specialization can also provide comfort and career satisfaction to practitioners, particularly those whose natural inclination is to develop a deep understanding in a narrow area of interest rather than broader expertise spanning multiple areas of interest. This focus on specific areas of medicine also provides a basis for broadening the understanding of key problems and research into solutions.

Doctor Stories—Practice Diversity

A less apparent and less widely acknowledged impact of specialization is that it requires a much more diverse workforce to fill these vastly different roles. To illustrate this, let's consider a sampling of roles, all filled by people we consider "doctors" but who may, on further examination, reveal themselves to only have this same title and little else in common.

Consider my friend Walt, a family physician who practices in a small community in Eastern Ontario. He attended medical school about 25 years ago and then entered a period of practical training that was available at that time called a rotating internship. Undertaken in a large urban hospital, it consisted of a year providing care under the supervision of fully qualified physicians in a number of settings, including emergency medicine, medical ward service, surgery, and obstetrics. Then, he moved to a small town and, for over 20 years, has been providing care to a group of individuals living in that community. Those people regard him as "their doctor." If they develop a health problem, they see Walt. He sees babies, children, young folks, and seniors. He sees people of all genders, sexual orientation, and socioeconomic status. He sees individuals and extended families. He sees essentially anyone who comes his way. He also takes a turn staffing the emergency department of the small local hospital and delivers babies born to women in his practice. Walt has developed several preventative programs that he provides for patients in his practice. He's an active member of the community, in which he and his wife have raised their own children and plan to retire.

Consider Carol, an ophthalmologist who, after medical school, undertook many years of training to not only qualify in that specialty, but also learn the latest techniques and approaches to patients with cataracts. Carol is highly proficient and provides care for the growing population of people with this condition. She is aware of the most modern approaches to this problem and is able to provide them skillfully and effectively. She has an approach that is consistent and effective for every patient. She helps them understand their problem, presents options, and guides them through the treatment process and recovery. She only sees patients who have that particular problem and treats them only until it is resolved to the extent that her skills and technology allow. She does not enquire or venture into patient issues or concerns that do not directly impact her ability to deal with patients' cataracts.

Finally, consider my friend John, a pathologist who is specialized in the neurologic system. John provides both general pathology services in a large urban hospital and is the resident expert on matters of neuropathology. John never sees a live patient, but his services are essential to the care of the people in his community. He is highly respected within the medical community and does research for which he's funded and regularly published. He teaches at the medical school affiliated with his hospital and is a popular teacher and mentor to students.

Walt, Carol, and John all provide valuable service to their communities, but services that vary markedly in character, scope, duration and setting. Importantly, Walt, Carol and John are themselves very different people with differing interests, strengths, and preferences. Remarkably, they are all members of the same profession and carry the same title—they are all medical doctors. They all underwent the same fundamental medical education. They were all admitted to medicine with the same process and criteria, and yet their professional lives are remarkably diverse.

Given the funding models described previously, their incomes will also vary considerably. Carol's professional income generated by doing ophthalmologic procedures may be several times that of Walt, who sees and assesses thirty to forty patients a day of all ages and with unclear or undetected problems. Although Carol's training took considerably longer than Walt's, this is nonetheless seen as fundamentally unjust by many and is a major source of friction within the profession.

And so, specialization can be seen as a natural evolution that has followed from the growth of knowledge and skills and has undoubtedly led to better care and outcomes for patients. But how has it affected family medicine, which remains rooted in the provision of generalist, holistic care to people of all types coming forward with as yet undiagnosed problems?

In the next chapter, we'll further explore this concept of "generalism," which is central to understanding the unique contributions and demands of family medicine.

CHAPTER SIX

The Challenges of Generalism

I ENTERED MEDICAL SCHOOL WITH THE intention to become a family physician in a small community. I qualified as such, but never did engage that sort of practice. Instead, I went on to specialize in a particular area of medicine, cardiology, to the full extent of training was possible at that time. Over the course of my career, my specialty has evolved such that many of the skills inherent to it have become sub-specialties, and even sub-sub-specialties of their own, to the point that almost everyone who enters my specialty engages up to three years of additional training to acquire those skills. I have become, in the later years of my career, a "generalist" within my specialty, because my practice involves people with much less differentiated problems, who often require multiple assessments and continuing care. I have come full circle or, more accurately, the world has evolved around me and left me (happily, I might add) no longer perceived as a "specialist," but as a "generalist."

Defining Generalism

Much has been written and definitions have been proposed. I favor two concepts that come from the British literature on the topic. One focuses on the breadth of interest and makes the point that the generalist, in distinction to the true "specialist" views health in a broader, unconstrained fashion.

> *"The essential quality is that the generalist sees health and ill-health in the context of people's wider lives, recognising and accepting wide variation in the way those lives are lived, and in the context of the whole person."*[9]

The second key concept is that the care provided by the generalist is deeply rooted in an empathic relationship that must exist between patient and physician. It is only in the context of such a relationship that medical conditions can be fully understood and treated.

> *"… establishing a rapport that can be therapeutic, in the sense of developing shared insights. It is enabling and developmental, in that it has the potential to move individuals on from where they are, whether this is in terms of understanding/knowledge, emotional capabilities, or in making decisions about undergoing investigations and treatment options."*[10]

Simply put, the primary interest of the generalist is the patient, not the medical condition. The generalist engages the patient as an

---

[9] Commission on Generalism. (2011). *Guiding patients through complexity: Modern medical generalism.* London: Royal College of General Practitioners and the Health Foundation. Retrieved from http://www.rcgp.org.uk/policy/commissn_on_generalsm.aspx

[10] Royal College of General Practitioners. (2012). *Medical generalism: Why expertise in whole person medicine matters.* London: Royal College of General Practitioners.

individual suffering from one or many conditions or personal circumstances. Those conditions may relate to discrete medical conditions, or broader personal and social issues. The generalist endeavors to develop a personal relationship, based on trust and confidence that will allow the patient to fully share all aspects of their lives, allowing full understanding of cause and paving the way to effective therapeutic interventions.

Characteristics of Generalist Practice

Given this conceptual understanding, we can describe in more pragmatic terms what truly entails a generalist medical practice. It boils down to three fundamental tenets:

1. The generalist approach is **holistic**. The generalist is interested in, and becomes involved with, the whole person. There are no pre-set limits or conditions that stand between patients and the generalist physician. The generalist engages patients whose problems are undefined and undifferentiated. For a generalist serving a particular community or population, anyone within that grouping is welcome.
2. The generalist approach is necessarily **comprehensive**. The generalist interest is determined by patient need and must therefore follow wherever those needs may lead. Although medical care has become increasingly compartmentalized to provide efficient application of expanding therapeutics, the generalist must be able to access and retain their role as the patient navigates those treatments.
3. The generalist approach is **continuing**. The generalist does not disengage when the patient completes a particular course of treatment, when treatment options fail, when no curative treatments are available, or when patients reach arbitrary age limits. The generalist follows the patient, not the disease.

Generalism within Various Specialites

Given the above definitions and characteristics, it becomes apparent that several medical specialties practice components of generalism. Emergency Medicine physicians and General Pediatricians, for example, engage people with completely undifferentiated and undefined problems. Psychiatrists must take a holistic approach to fully grasp all aspects of their patient's illness in order to establish working diagnoses. Medical sub-specialists who follow patients with chronic cardiac, renal, or arthritic disease, for example, must provide continuing care, often engaging co-existing conditions that may arise.

It can also be said that any physician (even a cardiologist) can choose to apply principles of generalism within the application of their chosen specialty. In fact, many would argue (in my opinion very effectively) that optimal care can only be truly provided in the context of that holistic approach and fully engaged patient-physician relationship.

However, family medicine is unique in that it provides all aspects of generalism as its core value proposition. In fact, the Canadian College of Family Physicians has clearly engaged generalism as its mission, well articulated in the Family Medicine Professional Profile:[11]

> *"Working together, family physicians provide a system of front-line health care that is accessible, high-quality, comprehensive, and continuous."*

That commitment is perhaps best expressed in the following quotation from Dr. Ian McWhinney, which featured prominently in

---

[11] College of Family Physicians of Canada. (2018). *Family Medicine Professional Profile*. Mississauga, ON: College of Family Physicians of Canada.

another recent publication from the CCFP outlining its educational objectives.[12] Dr. McWhinney was a British-born physician and academic who practiced and taught in Ontario for many years becoming known as the "founding father of family medicine" in Canada.

> *"If we (family physicians) are to fill our place, it is crucial that our commitment be unconditional: patients should feel confident that they will never be told, 'This is not my field.'"*

The Professional Challenges of Generalism

Several years ago, I attended a retirement dinner given to honor a longstanding and widely respected family doctor. At one point in the evening, I had an opportunity to chat with him and asked what he considered to be the biggest change in the world of medicine since he began practice many years ago. He surprised me by saying he didn't think much had really changed. Perhaps sensing my astonishment, he went on to explain that certainly the technology and range of therapeutics had evolved… *"but the patients show up with the same problems they've always had. They hurt, can't breathe, can't walk, can't cope…the list of things you have to deal with is the same list it's always been. Oh, we have more diagnoses to make and many more therapies to use, but they're the same people with the same problems as when I started."*

Indeed, my friend reminded me that the fundamental issues that afflict human beings and cause them to seek help from medical doctors are limited and unchanging. We call these issues "symptoms" or, more broadly in the medical world, "clinical presentations." These are

---

[12] Fowler, N., Oandasan, I., & Wyman, R. (Eds.). (2022). *Preparing our Future Family Physicians: An Educational Prescription for Strengthening Health Care in Changing Times*. Mississauga, ON: College of Family Physicians of Canada.

the constellation of sensations and physical changes that are the lived manifestations of disease states. The challenge of clinical medicine is to detect and assess these symptoms and signs so that their underlying triggering disease can be defined. We call this process *diagnosis*. Therapies to treat or cure (*therapeutics*) can only be effectively applied after a diagnosis is established. The Medical Council of Canada, in the process of defining objectives for its examinations, has defined about 120 of these presentations, and they form the basis for medical school teaching. They don't change because the human body hasn't fundamentally changed with respect to how it responds to various injuries and diseases.

For example, one of these presentations is dyspnea, or shortness of breath. People have been experiencing shortness of breath as a manifestation of injury or disease since the first human progenitor walked upright. There are many conditions (pulmonic, cardiac, hematologic, traumatic, infectious, congenital) that can cause it, and that list grows as new pathogenic processes (such as COVID-19) emerge. The medical doctor's diagnostic challenge is to uncover the precise cause through a detective-like process that involves listening carefully to the account of how it has affected the patient (everyone being an individual, with a nuanced experience) and examining the patient to detect signs that may be a clue to cause. The more precise and accurate the diagnosis, the more effective the therapies that can be applied.

Specialties differ with respect to the spectrum of presentations they deal with, and the depth to which they engage therapeutics. The more highly specialized these disciplines are, the narrower the scope and greater the extent to which they are involved in therapeutics, particularly interventions such as surgery.

Family medicine, with its generalist and comprehensive scope, has no such restriction as to the number of presentations they might encounter. Family physicians must therefore be prepared to engage patients with *any* clinical presentation. The major challenge is to establish diagnoses and determine a therapeutic path.

In the early days of medicine, when therapies were very limited, it was practical to expect that a single physician would be capable of providing whatever therapies were available. As medical knowledge and therapeutics have expanded to a remarkable degree, that expectation is no longer reasonable. In fact, that's why so many specialties have emerged—to provide a workforce to share that load, particularly the therapeutic components. The new discipline that has emerged is one of *consultancy*, where various specialists are called upon to provide guidance or assume components of care when required.

That process, however, begins with an assessment by a generalist (usually a family physician) who assesses the patient and establishes a diagnosis.

What's obvious from all this is that family medicine is, for most patients, the critical entry point to medical care. For many, it may be the only encounter they require to resolve their issue. But, for most, further assessment and therapy may be required from a physician with more focused expertise. Family medicine is not only essential, but also highly demanding. The family doctor must be a highly skilled diagnostician, which is greatly aided by having established a relationship with the patient that allows for full understanding of their circumstances, and an unfettered sharing of information based on a bedrock of mutual trust. It's also clear that to be fully effective the family doctor must have full access to those other specialists who will provide complementary care if and when required. All those components are essential to the provision of optimal patient care.

The Personal Challenges of Generalism

> *"Would you rather know something about everything, or everything about something?"*

This quotation from one of my former teachers sums up elegantly the essential difference between generalist and more highly specialized disciplines. Generalists have broad interests and a drive to explore every aspect of medical care. They resist confinement to a single domain. The more highly specialized doctor is much more comfortable working within pre-defined boundaries and developing what might be considered deeper and more complete understanding. In the end, there is plenty of room and need for both, but there are some realities that the generalist family doctor will face in the course of their work:

1. They will inevitably uncover and define problems for which they will not be able to provide full care.
2. They will, for those patients, need to ask for the help of other specialists.
3. Although their role is critical, it may be overshadowed by the specialist(s) who provides the key therapeutic intervention.

To illustrate, consider again the example of Sara related in Chapter 1. Sara received excellent care from dozens of doctors and other providers in the course of her long illness and recovery. However, none of it would have occurred, and she would not have survived, if not for the concern, diagnostic skills, and persistence of Rachel, the family doctor who encountered her for the first time in the walk-in clinic. Rachel is the true hero of the story. And yet, her role may not be recognized as such by those involved, even by Sara and her family.

Family doctors must be people who are able to take deep personal satisfaction in a role that brings great benefit, but not the recognition it deserves. They are the embodiment of the so-called Fifth Business, (the phrase made famous by the book of the same name by Robertson Davies)—they orchestrate the play and go unnoticed by the audience and, often, by the actors on the main stage. They must be people who have the humility to admit to their limitations and seek help when needed. They must find fulfillment and personal validation in the knowledge that they have provided valuable service, even in the absence of external acknowledgement.

This can only happen if their motivation extends beyond personal goals. They must be truly dedicated to the service of the patients they encounter. The effective and personally fulfilled family doctor is, first and foremost, a selfless individual truly dedicated to the service of others.

Money and Other Vexing Issues

Although all medical specialties encounter difficult challenges these days, there are some that particularly impact generalist specialties, and family medicine in particular.

The requirement for space and staff

Many specialties require the use of hospital-based resources and spaces. Although this limits access and imposes considerable bureaucratic challenges, those who practice in these fields do not have the financial and administrative obligation to support the resources required.

Generalist specialties such as family medicine are largely practiced in privately operated offices and clinics. Those physicians are therefore required to financially support and administratively manage such facilities. This imposes obligations and stresses which require considerable attention and diverts time and attention from their intended work. Moreover, these obligations extend far beyond their training or natural inclinations.

In the words of many family doctors, "I didn't go to medical school to become a business manager." And the public would be alarmed to learn how much time this siphons away from the care these doctors are able to provide to their patients.

Inequitable payment schemes

Most doctors in Canada are paid based on the "fee for service" (FFS) billing. Although many, particularly family physicians, have engaged models that provide some form of global reimbursement for services, the principles underlying the establishment of those payment and their ongoing assessment are based on FFS "marketplace" equivalencies.

In the FFS model, doctors are paid based on each individual service they provide. All physician-related activities are listed, and each assigned a fee. When physician services were simple, basically consisting of visits, this was straightforward. However, as physician-related services grew more diverse with the expansion of procedures, diagnostic services, various types of visits ranging from routine to urgent, from the simple to complex, and potentially occurring any time of day or night, the number and types of fees expanded dramatically. In Ontario, the FFS schedule of benefits is now 970 pages long and includes several thousand potential codes. The preamble alone is 120 pages.

A fundamental problem with the FFS concept is that it has evolved with no clear rationale as to how fees are provided as new codes have been added, as a result strongly favoring therapeutic interventions over diagnostic services. More about all this comes in the next chapter but, as an illustrative example, let's return again to Sara's story from Chapter 1. For the urgent care assessment where Sara's problems were defined and several calls were made to get the process underway that eventually led to her recovery, the family doctor would likely have received about $80. Almost everyone subsequently involved in her care would have been paid considerably more, some up to twenty times more. Without minimizing the value of all those critical specialist interventions, none could have occurred without the initial assessment and key insights provided by the family physician. What's the relative worth of each health care provider? Whatever one's philosophy about their relative value, the result is that family doctors are among the lowest paid of all physicians, even before practice expenses are considered.

And to make matters worse, family physicians face the disproportionate expenses related to their practice setting. Specialists who are procedurally or in-patient based, and who work in hospitals, aren't responsible for maintaining the premises, equipment, or for supporting the other key staff involved in their work. Family doctors, in sharp contrast, largely work in office settings and are personally responsible for finding and maintaining site and equipment, and for hiring and paying support personnel. These costs cut into personal income, which is particularly galling since family doctors already have less gross income potential than procedurally or institutionally based specialties. It also demands a burden for business acumen and management skill, which is not part of their training or inherent interest. Unlike a sole practitioner lawyer, who can readily increase her hourly rate to cover her overhead and related costs, the family doctor is beholden to the government fee schedule. Family doctors therefore exist in a liminal state: they are forced to be exemplary business managers yet are restricted from enjoying the basic flexibility afforded to other small businesses.

The burden of "paperwork"

The advent of electronic medical records (EMRs) should, in principle, allow for better access and confidentiality. However, much of the key information must be entered directly by physicians. This has demanded a major time commitment for family doctors, particularly in office-based practices. It's estimated that family doctors may be spending up to a quarter of their time typing information into their computers or extending their workday well into the evenings and weekends.

In addition, the number and complexity of the forms (insurance, health reports, licensing) that require physician completion have been steadily increasing.

All this clerical activity expected of family physicians is stealing time that could be spent with patients, adding to their frustration with the role, and is no doubt a deterrence to the career choice and a significant contributor to decisions to change careers altogether.

Underappreciation of the role

There is a moment after a long and difficult surgical procedure when the surgeon, still dressed in surgical scrubs and obviously fatigued, can come to a waiting room full of anxious family members and say to them: "The surgery went well. We were able to accomplish everything we set out to do. I think we're going to be fine." In that moment, the surgeon is seen as a conquering hero. And deservedly so. They have provided invaluable service.

There are no such moments for family doctors.

And yet, such successful surgeries may never have occurred if not for the early intervention of a family doctor.

Summarizing

Generalist medical specialties, and family medicine in particular:

- Are essential to the delivery of optimal medical care.
- Are essential to the overall functioning of the health care system.
- Are highly demanding professionally.
- Require special personal attributes and high levels of dedication.
- Are burdened with high requirements for practice management and clerical expectations.
- Are among the most poorly compensated medical specialties.

So, how does all this come about? Certainly, the system was not primarily designed to impose such inequities. It has, nonetheless, evolved in a manner that imposes unintended and damaging consequences. In the next chapter, we'll explore in more detail how the current system plays out for those involved.

CHAPTER SEVEN

The Elephant in the Room

WE'VE ALLUDED IN PREVIOUS CHAPTERS to instances where the compensation received for various services seemed misaligned to their positive impact on patient care.

In Chapter 1, the doctor who looked after Sara in the after-hours clinic and was so essential to assessing her condition and getting the process of treatment underway was paid much less than the various doctors who were involved in specific aspects of her care once the diagnosis had been made.

In Chapter 5, we learned that not only income, but practice settings and costs varied considerably across various medical specialties.

Let's explore this a little further.

Melissa's Story

Melissa was overjoyed to learn she'd been accepted to medical school. As the daughter of a schoolteacher and retail store operator, she developed the image of a doctor's life based on her encounters with the family physician she'd seen for various minor childhood ailments and other doctors who lived and worked in the small community that was home to Melissa and her family. She was intrigued by a family doctor's potential to beneficially impact lives and was always an eager and capable learner with particular interest in the sciences. It seemed a natural fit.

Melissa never gave much thought to how she'd be paid as a doctor. She knew, of course, that doctors were paid well, but had no real concept of how much, or how it was provided.

In her final year of medical school, Melissa and a group of her peers met with a senior physician for a seminar on "the business of medicine". She was surprised to learn that, for most doctors, there is no regular pay check, no contract, and no package of benefits. She came to learn that most doctors are reimbursed not like her schoolteacher mother, but much more like her retail businessman father. Most doctors, she learned, operated their practices as small businesses with expenses and payrolls to maintain and had concerns very similar to those she recalls her father was struggling with. The income of their practice, in Canadian provinces, derived exclusively from something called the Schedule of Benefits (or, colloquially, the fee schedule) which was several hundred pages long and listed several thousand separate and finely detailed services covering anything any doctor might provide to any patient. Each item was associated with a fee payable to the doctor providing it, which had apparently been vigorously negotiated between an organization representing doctors and the government responsible for dispensing taxpayer-generated revenues for those services. The doctor's job was therefore to select the appropriate fees that applied to each patient encounter and submit the fees for reimbursement. When Melissa reviewed the items, she was struck by the sheer volume of fee codes available, the degree of detail provided for each, and the apparent randomness of the fees associated. She was assured by the instructor that, with practice, she'd become comfortable with the process, but would need to develop familiarity and skill with the fee schedule in order to ensure she "maximized her billing potential." Was she now, unsuspectingly, just like her retail businessman father who, amid her schooling, warned her of the risks and burdens of running a business?

Melissa, who had never regarded her patients as opportunities for "billing potential," found this whole exercise confusing and profoundly discouraging. For the first time, she questioned her career decision.

Liam's Story

Liam graduated from medical school five years ago. He completed a three-year residency in internal medicine and was then accepted into a cardiology program. He and his wife have two small children and a large debt accumulated in the course of his education. They've only been able to repay a small amount of that since his graduation.

Becoming a cardiologist has been Liam's dream for many years, dating back to undergraduate work he did in physiology. He is very happy with the program and his role in it. He has been particularly interested in the treatment of patients with heart failure, which has become a subspecialty within the field. He's taken an active interest and even been involved in the publication of three papers on the subject. He recognizes that there is a great need for more targeted assessment and treatment of these patients. He would like to do even more training in heart failure and eventually set up a heart failure service in a university center. However, he's found during his training that this plan would have significant financial implications. He's learned that cardiologists provide a wide variety of diagnostic and therapeutic procedures, each of which is "billed" individually and rather lucratively. These are all provided in addition to the basic patient assessment fee and can increase overall income greatly. In fact, for most cardiologists, a day spent doing procedures or interpreting tests pays far more than the time spent seeing patients directly in the clinic or office. However, there is no such increased billing associated with the management of heart failure patients. Consequently, if he chooses to pursue a career in heart failure, he will work just as hard but be paid much less than his colleagues who engage in other areas of interest.

Let's take a closer look at the system that gives rise to these and other problems that can compromise patient care and the trust they have in their doctors.

How Doctors Are Paid

So, how do doctors get paid, precisely? In the medical context, there are several models by which doctors are paid for being doctors:

In the **fee-for-service model**, doctors are paid based on each individual service they provide. All physician-related activities are listed, with each assigned a fee. When physician services were simple, basically consisting of visits, this was straightforward. However, as physician-related services became more diverse with the expansion of procedures—diagnostic services, plus various types of visits ranging in urgency and complexity, and potentially occurring any time of day or night were now the norm—the number and types of fees expanded dramatically.

In the **capitation model**, doctors are provided a set fee for each patient they take into their practice. The fee is consistent regardless of patient circumstances and is intended to cover all services that might be required to care for that patient. This model is commonly used in family medicine practices where physicians "roster" patients and receive an annual payment based on that number.

As **salaried employees**, doctors are paid a fee to fulfill certain responsibilities, which usually involve aspects of patient care, but may involve other responsibilities as well. A hospital, for example, might engage a qualified physician to provide care for patients admitted to a particular ward of the hospital. The physician would be expected to ensure high standards of care provided in an efficient manner, but there would be no specific expectations of the number of visits or procedures provided. If it is a teaching hospital (i.e., affiliated with a medical school), the physician might have additional administrative or teaching responsibilities as well.

Alternative funding plans are models of care by which groups of physicians are contracted by a government ministry or local health authority to provide an agreed-upon spectrum of services for a negotiated fee. The doctors involved in the plan determine collectively how the funding is to be distributed among them.

If we could draw an analogy to how communities pay for fire services, salary arrangements are like paying firemen for being firemen within a community and taking care of any fire-related issue that arises. As such, they are expected not only to deal with fire emergencies but also to prevent fires, train new firemen or volunteers, and be continuously available. They are regarded as the community experts with respect to fire prevention and suppression, plus they guide government policy and perhaps even advance research into more effective approaches to fighting fires. Their goals are defined as high-level issues such as public safety and prevention. Their success is measured in terms of lives saved, personal injuries averted, and fire-related property damage prevented. And so, a reduced number of fires would be an index of success. Such a system requires a considerable degree of trust between the community and the firefighting profession because success in reducing the number of fires could be interpreted as less need for firemen. In other words, they could be working to promote their own obsolescence. It also requires some assessment of the value of firemen, but that assessment would be based on a broad view of skills and knowledge, far beyond simply extinguishing fires.

Capitation would be like paying a flat fee for any fires that arose, regardless of whether they are towering infernos or small backyard barbeque mishaps. Payment becomes a simple calculation based on the number of blazes squelched, regardless of size, and based on a previously negotiated, agreed-upon average fee. This would be effective in ensuring responsiveness to emergencies but ignores the preventative aspects of fire management and control and could result in underfunding from year to year. It does not provide for the provision of community expertise or consultation on policy issues and requires a periodic negotiation that will focus not on community goals, but on the economic interests of firemen versus those of the community.

Fee-for-service is like paying for each component of any potential fireman-related activity individually. It would require setting separate fees for any service that could potentially arise, including:

- Getting into equipment
- Driving the truck (and how far)
- Putting up the ladder
- Climbing the ladder (by the rung)
- Rescuing people (by number, and weight)
- Operating the hose
- Resuscitation
- Evaluating the damage (by the hour)

Clearly this would require an exhaustive and complex list of potential services that would need to be re-assessed regularly as technology and public expectations of fire management evolved. Negotiations regarding what's included and how much reimbursement is provided for each would be contentious and would pit the personal interests of the firefighters against the impact on societal resources and other needed services. It's easy to imagine that simply maintaining and administrating such an inventory would become a major industry in itself and that these negotiations would stray far from any focus on public safety.

Most physician payments in Canada are provided based on the fee-for-service approach. In Ontario, the Schedule of Benefits lists all fees payable to physicians through the Ontario Health Insurance Plan, which is, as previously noted, an exhaustively long list of "billable" services that has evolved over the years as diagnostics and therapeutic options have emerged. The effect has been that more recent entries are valued more highly because longstanding items (such as fundamental patient assessment) have been held relatively steady to lessen overall impact. As a result, procedural work is much better compensated than are personal patient encounters and assessments. A day spent engaged in a series of surgical procedures, administering anesthetics, or interpreting diagnostic studies is therefore much more lucrative than a day scheduled seeing patients in a clinic and understanding the full panoply of their needs.

In addition, there is little provision for the costs associated with the generation of those fees. Doctors operating within their own office or clinic facilities will therefore have overhead expenses that would not be the case for those who are able to generate fees within a hospital or other publicly funded facility.

All this means that family medicine suffers from a double whammy in the FFS model, of having very few procedural fees available on the one hand, while usually incurring more overhead expenses on the other, as Melissa and Liam have learned.

Capitation and salary compensation models certainly have the potential to address these discrepancies. But as we shall explore later, solving the payment gap problem gets at a symptom, but not at the root cause of our family physician shortage problem and physician ennui problem.

Finally, and perhaps most significantly, the methods we choose to compensate physicians also express, intentionally or not, the extent to which we value the service they provide.

President Joe Biden is fond of the following statement which he's made numerous times, including while introducing a recent federal budget:

> *"Don't tell me what you value, show me your budget, and I'll tell you what you value."*

It's typically pithy, direct, and relevant to this issue of physician compensation. We may profess to value direct patient interaction, prevention, and ongoing monitoring, but if we pay ten to twenty times more for time spent doing a procedure than for the initial assessment, counseling and preparation of the patient for that procedure, what are we in fact saying?

So, given all these considerations, can such folks be found and recruited into the profession? The answer to that starts with an examination of how and why young people presently enter the profession of family medicine.

CHAPTER EIGHT

Who Becomes a Doctor?

Caitlyn's Story

CAITLYN IS IN THIRD YEAR at university. She has been actively planning her medical school application since Grade 10. Strongly supported by her parents, she has researched and studied the application process and made a list of things she feels she needs to achieve to optimize her chances of success. Over the years, she has been slowly and deliberately addressing each item.

Knowing that academic success is essential to ensure acceptance to medical school, she has devoted herself to her studies. In high school, she would study long hours and become very upset on the rare occasions that she achieved less than 90 percent on a test, exam, or assignment. Each year, she finished at the top of her class and received academic awards.

She undertook numerous volunteer opportunities in health care settings, reasoning that this would demonstrate, to an admissions committee, her commitment to a medical career. She found these opportunities were widely sought after and hard to come by but, with the support of her parents and family friends, she was able to volunteer at a local nursing home and hospital.

Through her high school science teacher and friend of her mother, she was also able to volunteer in a research project carried out at the local hospital. Although her duties were restricted to greeting volunteer study participants and ensuring forms were completed, she was able to make contacts with the doctors involved and learn about how the research was conducted. Those doctors agreed to write letters of reference attesting to her reliability and interests in research.

She learned that participation in team sports was valued by many medical school admissions committees. Although not athletically inclined, she joined the field hockey team and devoted herself to practice and improvement. Her commitment was lauded by the coach, and she was eventually made a co-captain of the team.

Her volunteer work and studies left little time for other endeavors or for a social life. Although she maintained friendships with a small group of classmates with similar interests and goals, there was no time for parties, boyfriends, or traditional summer jobs in customer service.

While selecting a university, she received many scholarship offers. Her choice was based, after careful study, on the reputation and ranking of the medical school at each institution.

She chose a university program in health sciences that she felt would best position her for her medical school application. This approach was based on studying the published rates of acceptance into medical school by graduates of that program. The more selective, the better.

At the university, she found student groups that provided mutual support for medical school application. These "pre-med" groups shared information about the application process and even invited speakers who provided insights and advice about strategies for acceptance.

In choosing the electives, she selected courses in which she would be most likely to achieve very high marks. She learned, for example, that in English and philosophy courses, scoring more than 90 was very rare, whereas it was much more likely to achieve such marks in certain science or math courses.

She knew that she would have to do very well in the Medical College Application Test (MCAT). She began preparing for it a year in advance, initially by purchasing two or three of the many books and practice tests available. She also found a two-week preparatory course that advertised an excellent record of success which she could take during the summer. Although it was expensive and required her to travel to another city, her parents were very willing to support her, paying for the course and the examination itself. When she finally took the exam, she did well above the average but felt she could improve further so she took it a second time the following summer after another prep course, improving her results slightly.

Caitlyn is also aware that various interviews will be required as a component of the application process. She is naturally quite nervous and uncomfortable about being put on the spot. Aware of this, she and her parents identified agencies that provide individualized counseling and support for students navigating the application process. They had contact with one agency that, for a substantial fee, assigned Caitlyn to a personal counselor, a successful medical student applicant.

Caitlyn has obviously strategized carefully and applied herself diligently to achieve her goal. She and her parents have sacrificed to a considerable degree. She has made key strategic choices and has an excellent chance of achieving her goal of entering medical school. But do Caitlyn's efforts prepare her for the life's work that she's chosen? Do her efforts and education to date prepare her for or even allow her to fully understand the nature of that life's work? And, relevant to the theme of this book, when faced with the choice, is Caitlyn likely to choose to become a family physician providing comprehensive and continuing care?

To begin to answer these key questions, let's explore the realities of the process she's engaging.

The Medical School Application Process— Facts and Figures

Almost all (98%) of students admitted to medical school graduate and become practicing doctors. Admission to medical school is, therefore, *de facto* admission to the profession.

The number of medical school positions in Canada is fixed by public authority. Medical education is expensive and largely subsidized by provincial governments, which therefore define the number of available seats in medical schools, based loosely on anticipated demands for physicians. These estimations have fluctuated in the past such that we have seen periods of both contraction and expansion.

Among Canadians, there is a very high demand for medical education. At Queen's University, about 6,000 applications are received for about 100 available positions each year. All Canadian schools receive many times more applications than they can accommodate. The hunger for a career in medicine is such that increasing numbers of Canadians are enrolling in medical schools in Australia, the Caribbean, Ireland, and in other countries, at considerable personal expenses and with no assurance of postgraduate training or eventual qualification to practice medicine in Canada. Although no accurate data is available, it's estimated that there are now more Canadians studying medicine outside Canada than within.

Medical schools are almost all university-based institutions with independent admission processes. In other words, they are free to set their own standards, admission criteria, and admission processes. Although the schools have good outreach practices to prospective candidates and meet to discuss and (to some extent) share practices, they are under no obligation to adhere to any centralized processes or principles in doing so.

Medical schools entrust the process to admissions committees. Within universities, the responsibility for medical school admissions is usually entrusted to a committee within the faculty of medicine or health sciences (as the case may be) and is largely separate from and independent of the general university admission process. The members of that committee are usually selected through a combination of appointments from the dean and election among faculty members. There are usually student members (who have themselves recently and successfully undertaken the admission process). Public members may be recruited, but there is no such obligation. The chair is appointed by and accountable to the dean and is usually a physician or basic scientist. Terms for members and chairs are time-limited and so there is rapid turnover, requiring much relearning of the complicated procedures and little opportunity for review or substantive reform. Accreditation standards require that a Canadian medical school "establishes and publishes admission requirements for potential applicants to the medical education program and uses effective policies and procedures for medical school selection, enrolment and assignment" but do not stipulate any linkage to societal needs or external accountability to address requirements for either the number or type of physicians they graduate.[13]

Medical schools place priorities on fairness, equity, and diversity in their application processes. Given the tremendous excess of applications for available seats, admission committees then face the enormous challenge of selecting the "most worthy" from so many worthy applicants. The challenge has been compared to trying to select which puppy to take home from a litter of adorable puppies. There is pressure, both real and perceived, to justify negative decisions.

---

[13] Committee for Accreditation of Canadian Medical School Standards and Elements. (2023). *Standards and elements* (Standard 10, p. 18).

Schools strive to ensure objectivity and fairness in their processes. They are therefore drawn to metrics that provide some basis for imagined objectivity. In addition, there has been mounting awareness in recent years of the importance of ensuring equitable access to groups previously underrepresented in medicine, including indigenous and racialized populations. Admission committees have undertaken significant measures to ensure equity in their processes, and most have established facilitated processes to ensure that specific targets for such historically underrepresented groups are achieved within admitting classes.

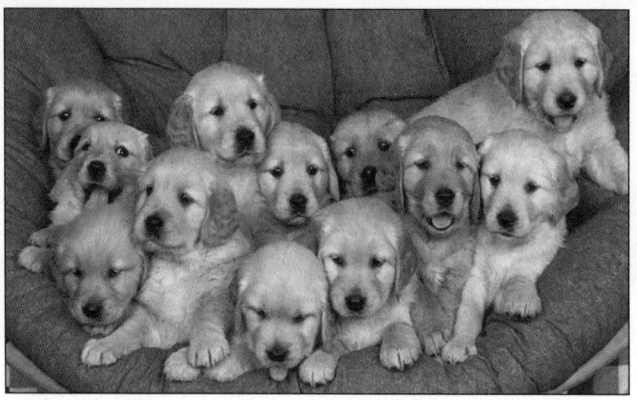

Retrieved from: https://www.animaroo.com/puppy-blog/pick-the-right-puppy-out-of-the-litter/

The two quantitative metrics most widely used are averaged grades obtained in university courses (Grade Point Average, or GPA) and results obtained in the MCAT. The MCAT is developed and administered by the Association of American Medical Colleges. It is provided at many sites across the United States and Canada multiple times per year. The current fee is US$325. Books and online material can be purchased to assist applicants in preparing for the exam. Also, many seminars, courses, and personal tutoring services are available at costs ranging up to several thousands of dollars. Most applicants will engage one or more of these preparatory options and will devote at least several months to preparation. Because most schools allow candidates to take the examination multiple times and accept the best results, many candidates undertake the preparatory process more than once.

Schools will ask applicants for an autobiographical sketch of some form, chronicling their academic and nonacademic activities. Although schools develop and safeguard their own criteria for assessing personal experiences, it's widely understood that most are looking for demonstrable evidence of community service, dedication and experience in health care delivery, research exposure, and a profile of nonacademic activity that would reflect qualities such as teamwork, leadership, motivation, and resilience.

Panel interviews and mini-medical interviews (MMIs) are being used increasingly by medical schools to better assess applicant's personal qualities. MMIs are short challenges where the candidate is expected to engage a particular problem or dilemma under observation. The intention is to assess the candidate's ability to engage a problem spontaneously, identify key issues, and communicate effectively. These are resource intensive and difficult to conduct and evaluate in a reliable manner. It's therefore not possible to apply such methods to a large number of applicants. Consequently, schools tend to use staged application processes that rely heavily on academic records and test metrics. In addition, since MMIs were introduced several years ago, awareness among the applicant population has risen leading to intense preparation and the emergence of many preparatory courses and even personal tutoring services, some of which advertise impressive "acceptance rates" among former clients. This all promotes a Hawthorne effect, whereby applicants alter their behavior to meet perceived expectations.

Applicants to Canadian medical schools are knowledgeable regarding the process and highly accomplished academically. Although little systematic data on the subject is available, it appears to all involved that the GPA and MCAT scores and personal experiences reported by applicants are increasing each year. Applicants understand the "system" and are highly strategic as they undertake their education and personal activities.

Back to Caitlyn

We have seen earlier how Caitlyn has done her homework, diligently researched the admission process, and carefully crafted her schoolwork and activities over the past several years to put herself in the best possible position for success. As a result, she has an excellent chance of being accepted to a medical school.

It's important to recognize that Caitlyn's story is not unusual or rare. In fact, it's likely that most successful applicants will relate very similar stories. Medical school applicants are informed, goal-oriented, driven individuals who are well supported, well financed, and able to devote extensive time and energy to this singular goal.

But, as one might expect given these accounts, there are prices to be paid for the practices that have emerged from this intensely competitive process. Let's consider some other experiences. Again, these are based on real people.

Miriam grew up in small community, part of a large family that had immigrated to Canada. She was always an excellent student but, largely for financial reasons, decided to attend a nearby college rather than university. She nonetheless was able to eventually study and become qualified as a clinical psychologist. For the past several years, she has been practicing in a mid-sized community, seeing patients referred for support by local family doctors. She also works closely with local social workers and with the only psychiatrist in the community. That psychiatrist is overwhelmed with referrals and has come to depend on Miriam to help manage the caseload. They've been discussing the possibility of Miriam becoming a psychiatrist. Both the psychiatrist and local medical community are very supportive of this.

When Miriam explores it further, she realizes the only option available to her is to apply to a medical school to obtain an MD degree and then apply to a five-year psychiatry program. She has to take the MCAT examination and hope that her marks are competitive with those of the myriad students applying directly from university programs. Even if she were able to gain admission, she doesn't feel she'd be able to afford to give up her salary and pay the tuition and expenses required. And it would be nine years before she'd achieved her goal.

And so, Miriam is essentially blocked from taking up a career that she's already very informed about and committed to, and for which her community has a desperate need.

Hassan grew up in a culturally and ethnically diverse section of a large city. He has recognized the barriers experienced by various ethnic groups for many years and feels very motivated to become a doctor to provide primary care in his home community. At university, he chooses to major in physics because it's always been an interest and he feels the analytical thinking will be an asset to his medical career. He does very well in his courses, achieving consistently well above average with marks in the mid- to upper 80s. However, his overall GPA is lower than that of most applicants for medical school who have undertaken programs where the average marks are much higher. After multiple attempts, and despite strong letters of support from community leaders and local physicians, he has been unsuccessful in getting an offer of admission.

In both cases, motivated and committed people who are very eager to provided much-needed services are essentially circumvented from doing so. Let's take a closer look at some of the unintended consequences of current admission practices.

Strategic selection of undergraduate courses and programs. Academic records have always been the cornerstone of the admission process. However, lack of uniformity regarding course content and evaluation rigor among institutions (and even departments in the same institutions) has eroded their reliability. It's widely appreciated that some universities and programs take pride in the demands they place on their students and the meaning of an honors grade. Students attending such institutions therefore put themselves at a competitive disadvantage, despite receiving what all would agree is an excellent educational experience. In addition, some disciplines, such as English and the humanities, rarely award marks above the low to mid-80s. Postgraduate science courses tend to award higher marks than undergraduate courses in the same discipline. Although all these vagaries are widely appreciated, there is no acceptable or fair means to equilibrate these inequities. Consequently, students interested in pursuing medical school admission may be making choices based on strategic priorities rather than interest or natural aptitude.

Résumé engineering. Applicants perceive a need to ensure their nonacademic résumés reflect interest in medical and humanitarian pursuits, and even research. Although such efforts are obviously laudable, they may be chosen for strategic rather than purely altruistic value and come with the price of exclusion from other healthy growth experiences. In addition, such experiences may not be equally available to applicants from diverse communities and socioeconomic backgrounds.

Commercialization of medical education. The large number of young people seeking admission to medical school has become an economic "market" with medical education being a "commodity." The cost of writing the MCAT (currently US$325) may not seem unreasonable but must be seen as part of a greater financial requirement in the aggregate, including costs of preparatory material, courses, travel to and from examination sites, and multiple examinations that many candidates undertake to ensure competitive results. University undergraduate courses in biologic sciences have increasingly taken on a distinctly "medical school prep" tone, to the point that program designations have evolved to terms that denote closer links to medical education ("health sciences" or "medical sciences"), even providing MCAT preparation as part of the curriculum and publishing statistics regarding the rate of medical school acceptance among enrolled students. Although such programs may be of intrinsic value, one wonders whether there is sufficient value and career opportunity for most participants in these programs who will not be successful in their medical school applications. Finally, the steadily increasing number of international medical schools that offer positions to students who are able to bear the financial burden and accept the uncertainties of postgraduate placement is a clear consequence of the mismatch between the demand and availability of medical school positions.

Premature exclusion (or selection) of medicine as a career option. Admission to medical schools is increasingly seen as the ultimate award for academic excellence. There is an emerging perception that only academically very successful students need apply and, conversely, that high academic success carries the expectation of medical school admission, almost as an earned right. Both perceptions are problematic. The former excludes (or at least fails to encourage) students based on very early and likely unrepresentative academic experiences. The latter runs the risk that students will set themselves, and parental expectations, on a determined career path with an incomplete understanding of the demands of that career or their own suitability. The embedded psychology of grades being determinative of ultimately being a good doctor becomes a kind of bean-counting exercise for aspiring doctors, in the same way that an historic perception of a good academic worthy of promotion (since abandoned in most graduate programs in North America) was solely one whose academic journal contributions were cited more often than their peers, irrespective of their teaching caliber or community impact in a chosen field of study.

Expense and sacrifice of other pursuits. The application process itself, the MCAT examination, MCAT preparation, and travel for interviews are all costs that applicants must bear. The process also requires *time*, which favors those who are able to take time away from summer or part-time jobs in order to study and travel. It also demands the tenacity, and income supports, to forgo other lucrative areas of study in terms of lifetime earnings potential available to these students with strong GPAs.

Favoring students from urban settings. This relates to the fact that students from rural areas must necessarily move away from home to attend university. In addition, volunteer opportunities, MCAT preparation courses, and the administration of the MCAT itself are much more available in urban centers. All of this is compounded by the fact that rural Canadians are known to have lower income than their urban counterparts.[14]

Socioeconomic status has an influence on individuals' perception of their suitability for medical school and a medical career. This is partially because students from more advantaged backgrounds have more access to role models in medicine and therefore more access to friends and family who "see them as a doctor" from a young age.[15] Students from higher income families receive more family and social encouragement to pursue medical education compared to those who self-identify as coming from "working-class" families.[15] The same study noted above about differences in role modeling for people with advantaged backgrounds also suggests that students from lower-income families are more likely to overestimate the costs,

---

[14] Greenhalgh, T., Seyan, K., & Boynton, P. (2004). "Not a university type": Focus group study of social class, ethnic, and sex differences in school pupils' perceptions about medical school. *BMJ, 328*(7455), 7455. Retrieved from https://doi.org/10.1136/bmj.328.7455.7455

[15] Beagan, B. (2005). Everyday classism in medical school: Experiencing marginality and resistance. *Medical Education, 39*(8), 777–784.

while simultaneously underestimating the financial benefits, of post-secondary education. They therefore encounter a narrative about earnings potential that runs counter to the one thrust upon their peers from more economically advantaged backgrounds.

It appears all this is having an effect. An important study by Irfan Dhalla and colleagues at the University of Toronto surveyed 1,223 first-year Canadian medical students and found that, compared to the general population, medical students were:

- Less likely to be of Black (1.2% vs 2.5%) or Aboriginal (0.7% vs. 4.5%) heritage
- Less likely to hail from rural areas (10.8% vs. 22.4%)
- More likely to have parents with master's or doctoral degrees (39.0% of fathers and 19.4% of mothers, compared to 6.6% and 3.0% respectively)
- More likely to have parents who were professionals or senior managers (69.3% of fathers and 48.7% of mothers compared to 12.0% of Canadians), including 15.6% of medical students having at least one physician parent.
- Less likely to come from households with incomes under $40,000 annually (15.4% vs. 39.7%)
- More likely to come from households with incomes over $150,000 (17.0% vs. 2.7%)[16]

The sacrifices that young people undertake to achieve medical school acceptance can have negative consequences for them. All young people must go through a process wherein they move away from the protection provided by parents, take on activities and pursuits of their own and begin to develop their own personal world

---

[16] Canadian Medical Association Journal. (2002). *CMAJ, 166*(8), 1029.

view and sense of identity. This process, referred to as individuation, typically occurs in the late teens and early twenties and, in North America, often plays out at colleges and universities. Yet, Caitlyn and young people like her devote themselves to their goals very early in life. They forgo many of the options and experiences that are critical to personal development. The decision to pursue a career in medicine can therefore prevent a young person from engaging valuable developmental experiences or from considering other interests and potential career options.

Beyond the simple issue of justice and fair treatment, and returning to our core theme of finding the family doctors we need, are these barriers disproportionately affecting applicants who might be predisposed to careers as the sort of family doctors that are so in demand?

Failure to Recognize Diverse Needs of Medical Specialties and the Disconnect between Physician Supply and Societal Needs

Let's recall the accounts of my friends Walt (the family physician), Amanda (the ophthalmologist), and John (the pathologist) recounted in Chapter 5. What's clear is that these are three very different people, with differing interests, strengths, and preferences. Nonetheless, they are all members of the same profession and carry the same title—they are all medical doctors. They all underwent the same fundamental medical education. They all entered medicine through the same admission process.

Despite this great role diversity, people continue to be selected for medical school (and effectively, to the profession) using a single point of entry. In other words, young people are accepted into the career in medicine without consideration of which of the more than 100 remarkably different career paths they will eventually pursue.

It is expected that they will learn about various specialties and decide what to pursue after they have already been accepted.

To help understand the impact of this single point of entry issue, let's consider the example of a large automobile manufacturer. The company produces a vast variety of models to address all needs of the driving public. They design, build, and sell all types of vehicles—large cars, small compact cars, sports cars, sports utility vessels, minivans, and trucks of all sizes from small pick-ups to large trucks that pull heavy trailers. To achieve this, they require a large and very diverse workforce that includes engineers, designers, draftsmen, assembly workers, advertising people, salespeople, clerical people, accountants, financial planners, and many more distinct and demanding roles.

Now imagine that the company has a hiring policy that is designed to seek out and hire talented and hard working folks who are passionate about the automobile industry in general but don't necessarily have any specific qualifications or interests. The plan is that those talented folks are raw material, or units of production, who will receive orientation and training after hiring. That training begins very general and becomes increasingly specialized based entirely on the evolving, self-guided interests of the new employee. How would such an organization function? How could it be assured of having enough people in each necessary role to meet its objective of providing sufficient automobiles of all varieties for the driving public? Clearly, it would be vulnerable to unpredictable surpluses and deficiencies in various areas of specialization needed. It would also be expending (and risking) considerable resources and time in training.

This is essentially the model that's currently used to provide for the diverse and increasingly complex medical needs of society. The car company, led by management, enjoys the agility to define and redefine a strategy on an annual or even quarterly basis that helps refine the type of personnel most oriented to accelerating the strategy.

Not so in medicine. There is no linkage between the current societal need for various types of physicians, and the process by which people enter the profession. In addition, as we've seen, there are aspects of the admission process that may be counterproductive to the recruitment of people likely to fill the pressing need for family physicians.

So, How Does All this Relate to Our Family Doctor Problem?

In the previous chapter, we reviewed the concept of the generalist practice and the qualities required of people who undertake those specialties.

All doctors, regardless of specialty, must combine an interest in the science of medicine with an ability and desire to engage people individually and as full and complex human beings as they come forward with their medical problems. However, those two interests don't always exist in similar proportions, nor does the inherent ability. For those who undertake truly generalist care, the interest in people tends to be the primary driver. They find fascination in exploring individual stories, in the global human experience, and take great satisfaction in exploring and clarifying the various nuances of those relationships. As described previously, they must also be people who are able to recognize their own limitations, engage other specialist colleagues as the need to do so inexorably arises, take satisfaction in the diagnostic process, and deal with the inherent uncertainty that can often accompany that pursuit. They must also be able to find personal fulfillment in the knowledge that they make key contributions to a patient's course, even when sometimes overshadowed by others who have engaged the therapeutic process after the difficult work of patient engagement and diagnosis has been completed. On a personal level, they must feel fulfilled knowing they've done a good job even if not acknowledged by others, even those who've benefitted from their work. *Internal validation* must suffice for these folks because *external validation* may be infrequent or nonexistent.

Does the admission process we have reviewed look for these special qualities essential to those destined to practice comprehensive, community-based family medicine?

Let's consider a side-by-side comparison:

Qualities favoring successful application for medical school admission	Qualities favoring a generalist specialty (particularly family medicine)
• Determination in pursuit of personal goals • Persistence • High academic achievement in scientific courses • Time and resources to prepare for entrance examinations • Time for and access to volunteer activities • Time for and access to research opportunities • Strong family encouragement and support	• Ability to form effective relationships with diverse individuals • Commitment to service • Ability to deal with uncertainty • Resilience • Integrity/trustworthiness • Community focus • Diligence • Maturity

The unfortunate reality is that these two sets of personal qualities do not align, nor should we expect them to. The good news is that, with a better understanding of the goals, processes, and tools currently available and widely used in the admissions processes, we can and should be able to better identify individuals much better suited for, and therefore more likely to engage in, the wondrous practice of family medicine that our entire health system depends upon.

CHAPTER NINE

The Long, Narrow Path

AS MENTIONED PREVIOUSLY, I WENT to medical school with an intention to become a family doctor. The plan was to eventually return to the small community in which I'd lived until moving away to attend university and to take over the practice of one of the several doctors who had lived out their careers providing medical care for people in that community. That was, after all, why one went to medical school. In fact, all my seventy-one classmates trained with the purpose of becoming what was described at the time as "general practitioners." That was the explicit objective of our four-year educational program and, with one further postgraduate year of practice preparation in any of a variety of different options provided and successful completion of a written examination, we were fully qualified and licensed to do so.

The world has changed rather dramatically over the past 40 years. Medical education, not so much.

The fundamental four-year (or in the case of some schools, three years concentrating the same basic content) primary medical education process is still in place. Its fundamental purpose remains to ensure applicants are educated and trained in all aspects of medical care. Since the early part of the 20th century, this fundamental education has been entrusted to universities. This came about substantially, but not entirely, because of a report on the state of existing medical education commissioned by the Carnegie Foundation for the Advancement of Teaching, carried out and published in 1911 by Abraham Flexner. In this landmark report, Flexner decried the lack of scientific and educational rigor in the teaching, provision of facilities, and qualifications of teaching faculty. He also questioned the financial conflicts inherent in payments going directly to those providing the teaching and also assessing the students. All this could be addressed by moving medical schools into universities where appropriate affiliations with teaching hospitals and oversight could be provided. And, indeed, it has for many decades.

That fundamental period of training ends formally with university graduation and bestowing a medical degree (the "MD"). It has become a rather coveted component in that "medical-doctoral" universities are considered a somewhat higher echelon in the world of postsecondary education. Such universities no doubt benefit reputationally, philanthropically, and practically by attracting the large number of young people wishing to enter medical school who hope that undertaking their undergraduate education at such an institution will enhance their chances of success.

However, the educational process that's required for eventual practice qualification has changed dramatically over the past several decades. In fact, people are far from qualified to practice at the time they complete medical school. The MD basically entitles them to enter one of about thirty "entry-level" specialties, some of which branch further into two or three years of specialization, resulting in about seventy potential specialties, one of which is family medicine (having transitioned from "general practice" with the advent of the College of Family Medicine, which outlines training requirements and examinations to ensure those requirements had been met).

For many, training doesn't stop there. As therapeutic options for many medical conditions have developed, areas of subspecialization have emerged in order to prepare doctors to provide them. In cardiology, for example, almost all who complete their three-year general cardiology training will choose to become an expert in a subspecialty, such as interventional (carrying out catheter based diagnostic and therapeutic procedures), electrophysiology (diagnosing and treating patients with heart rhythm problems), imaging, or heart failure. To obtain these enhanced skills, already fully trained and qualified physicians will seek out and undertake one, two or more years of additional training to become proficient in these fields. Assuming an undergraduate degree was completed before entering medical school, it can take up to 16 years from the time of entry to university to qualify fully in one of these fields. This is because additional training has always been considered as an add-on at the end of a period of training, with really no consideration as to whether all the training is truly required for that eventual role. The reality is many highly specialized doctors receive most of the training they will require to function within their specialty in the last two to three years of that journey. The rest is about getting to the finish line.

Family medicine officially requires two postgraduate years to qualify, but almost all students choose to undertake a third year to develop enhanced skills, and it appears most graduates choose to practice in those more restricted areas rather than taking on comprehensive and continuing care in a traditional office and hospital-based practice setting. In fact, at the time of this writing, the College of Family Medicine was close to the final approval of a recommendation to expand the training period to three years to accommodate this growing trend.

All this change has had serious consequences and impact on the training of community-based family doctors.

Losing the Numbers Game

No longer the only option available, family medicine competes for the attention of students and potential trainees amid a steadily growing number of options. Although medical school positions have expanded, they have not kept up with that expansion. For example, in the mid-20th century, a graduating medical class of fifty students would provide almost that number of family physicians. By the 1980s, when my class of 1970 graduated, about half, or thirty-five, entered that workforce. A contemporary graduating class at Queen's, for example, consists of about 100 students, with about a quarter of them entering family medicine training. Of those, at least half opt for an area of specialized interest or to provide intermittent relief care (locums), meaning that only about twelve undertake the sort of comprehensive, community-based care that is so desperately lacking. Although numbers and percentages vary, the same trends are occurring across the country. The numbers are going in the wrong direction.

University MD Programs Have an Identity Crisis

These university-based MD programs have as their core and stated purpose the general education of students to prepare them for any potential area of specialization. This means students require education and clinical exposure to all areas of practice, regardless of their eventual career track. For example, it's expected that all students will have hands-on experience with delivering a baby, performing pelvic examinations, and assisting surgical procedures despite the knowledge that, for most, those skills will never again be undertaken in their further training or careers. Further, those going into specialties where such skills are required will be doing them many times and under expert supervision during those residencies.

This mandate to provide everything for all necessarily places students in specialized practice settings, particularly hospitals, and under the supervision of non-family medicine specialists. As a result, students get little exposure to community-based family medicine and little opportunity to work alongside those who practice it in those settings.

The students, for their part, are very much focused on career exploration and the process of getting into specific residency programs after medical school. Because almost all of them are undecided about their specialty choice at the start, they are very eager to "sample" many specialties as if at a buffet, and, once decided on a path and location, their overwhelming attention becomes fixed on optimizing their chances of being accepted into that program. Many of these programs are very competitive, thus adding to the stress and distraction and essentially reactivating the same competitive juices and strategies that got them into medical school.

The Narrow Gate Issue

Here are a few facts:

- A medical degree is an absolute prerequisite to becoming a doctor in Canada
- Medical degrees in Canada are provided only at university-based medical schools
- Almost everyone (98 percent) who enters medical school graduates and practices medicine
- Universities, through their medical schools, have independent authority for setting admission standards and the practices and protocols of admission

As a result of all this, entry to the medical profession in Canada is effectively under the control of these university-based medical schools.

This is despite the fact that provincial governments fund substantial proportions of the education of medical students (far over and above individual tuition payments).

All this has critical implications relevant to the family medicine shortage because there is no requirement for those admission processes to be linked formally to societal needs, on the part of either the students being admitted or the school itself. There is a clear disconnect between the admission authority that resides at the level of the university and the needs of society.

There is also a more fundamental issue at play. Universities are, and should be, places where young people can come to learn and explore various areas of interest, grow as people, and hopefully settle on a life's work. Medical schools have always operated under this basic understanding, allowing students the space and options to explore and choose without restriction. Up until recent years, this process has, without interference, worked out. However, the current physician workforce crisis is forcing some critical questions. Are medical schools educational institutions that primarily serve the interests and aspirations of tuition-paying students, or are they public institutions that provide a critical workforce to serve the needs of society? If we were to ask the consumers of the products of medical school this question, how would they answer?

Given the importance of the crisis we're facing, and the fact that university-based medical schools essentially control the pipeline, this vexing question can no longer be ignored.

CHAPTER TEN

Who's Driving the Bus?

HAVING ESTABLISHED THAT THERE ARE structural and longstanding problems with the processes that select and train doctors and that these issues negatively impact the supply of family physicians, it seems reasonable to ask how this came about and how it might be addressed. To do so, it's necessary to examine further the steps required to become a doctor in Canada, and how each of them is controlled.

That process, for most who go on to practice medicine in this country, currently consists of at least four and (for most) up to six distinct steps or stages.

Stage 1—Getting into Medical School

The first stage in this process is getting into a medical school. Because it is mandatory to obtain a medical degree to engage in all aspects of medical training and qualification, this must be considered a necessary step along the way although it is not officially part of the educational process.

Over the last two decades, this process has become highly competitive. The ratio of applicants to available seats across Canada is approximately 30:1 and is as high as 60:1 at some schools. Importantly, the admission processes at each of the seventeen (soon to be twenty) Canadian medical schools, as we've seen, is the exclusive domain of the medical school itself and the university in which it is housed. The admission criteria, required submitted material to be considered, and the interview processes itself are all determined by committees established by the medical school. Those committees, composed largely of faculty members, agonize as they work to develop processes that will identify optimal candidates based on criteria they feel to be relevant. At the same time, they endeavor mightily to be fair to all applicants. Everyone recognizes they have far more qualified applicants than seats, and the overwhelming sentiment is to justify the large number of rejections.

Those processes tend to be heavily dependent on academic performance and the results of the MCAT. These criteria both establish academic aptitude and provide an objective numerical basis for decision-making. It's widely recognized that these metrics are somewhat effective in identifying academic success during medical school, but there is poor correlation with success in the clinical environment, and very little information about long-term career success or satisfaction.

Because of the competitive nature of the admission process, applicants begin planning and preparing early in life, often in early high school. A commercial industry has ballooned to assist applicants who are willing to purchase such services through the process.

It is recognized widely that the process imposes financial and social barriers on medical school access. It is also the impression of many involved in the process that the qualities and applicant attitudes selected are more likely to favor students predisposed to non-generalist specialties.

As noted, the process is controlled by the individual medical schools who certainly collaborate and share experiences with one another, but there is no centralized process nor universally accepted set of criteria or processes.

Medical school admissions are also highly influenced by accrediting bodies that enforce standards needing to be met with respect to the establishment of fair and objective committees and any avoidance of conflict of interest, but do not speak to the specific criteria or processes required. It should also be noted that many Canadians seek a medical education in foreign medical schools. The exact number is unclear, but it's widely felt that at least as many Canadians are attending medical school outside Canada as within. These international schools, of course, have their own criteria for admission and it must be acknowledged that they are often motivated by commercial interest.

Stage Two: Primary Medical Education

A medical degree is an absolute prerequisite for medical training and can only be obtained through enrolment in university-based medical degree programs. The so-called undergraduate medical education programs are usually four-year programs although two three-year programs exist in Canada and meet the same criteria and content requirements in a more concentrated curriculum. The primary purpose of these programs is to prepare students to engage any medical specialty. At the end of medical school, students apply to—and almost all are accepted into—one of about thirty primary medical specialty programs any of which may be provided in any of the medical schools across the country. There are about five hundred such programs to which students apply through a matching service that they engage at a cost. Acceptance into some of these programs is highly competitive. Family medicine is one of these thirty streams.

Medical schools are very much challenged to concurrently provide broad medical education that would allow candidates to enter any program while at the same time supporting students in the process of deciding upon a career track and then engaging that competitive process.

This phase of medical education is primarily controlled by university-based medical schools that are independently responsible for developing and delivering their curriculum. Accrediting bodies have a wide variety of standards that address requirements. The Medical Council of Canada has, for over 100 years, been providing a qualifying examination that medical students must pass at the end of medical school to engage in residency programs. The matching service that provides the mechanism by which students apply to postgraduate programs does not attempt to influence the criteria by which students are selected, but the application processes they establish are highly influential in determining student behavior and planning at the medical school level.

The various postgraduate programs across the country independently determine their own entry criteria and oversee their own processes. Medical student societies, which exist both at the national and provincial levels, are very well informed, very well organized, and highly motivated to review and influence the application process.

Medical school education is also influenced by provincial governments and ministries expressing strong views toward the selection processes and curricular content as they anticipate that medical schools in their province will provide them the best opportunity to ensure physicians are recruited to that province. Their policies tend to be based on short-term goals, which are difficult to reconcile with the medical education process; the education process clearly requires long-term forecasting in order to address systemic issues such as the shortage of family physicians. Those policies can also vary dramatically and unexpectedly as elections sprout up and as both political and administrative leadership changes.

Stage Three: Primary Residency

Specialty training programs (commonly referred to as the beginning of postgraduate medical education) cover about thirty entry-level disciplines and are provided across the country. Not all are provided at all seventeen medical schools and the distribution of positions varies somewhat year to year (based largely on provincial funding), but at any time, there are likely between 450 and 500 such programs. They are operated by clinical departments based in academic medical centers, staffed by university-appointed faculty. They function more-or-less independently with respect to the establishment and adjustment of curricula, clinical teaching placements, and assessment standards. Because the programs are largely conducted in hospital and clinical sites, these learners, who are now provisionally licensed within their province to practice in supervised settings, are paid employees as well as learners. The funding for their salaries comes from the provincial governments and is administered largely through the hospitals to which they are most closely affiliated. However, they will move between various teaching sites including community-based sites and clinical practice settings. This is particularly true for family medicine training programs.

Family medicine training programs are the largest of these and are provided at all medical schools and their distributed teaching sites. At any time, about 40 percent of learners at this level are enrolled in family medicine programs.

This stage of training is also highly influenced by the College of Family Physicians, which oversees family medicine training across the country, and the Royal College of Physicians and Surgeons, which sets standards for training and assessment in all the other specialties. The Royal College has established a large number of specialty committees for this purpose.

Learners at this level are all members of their provincial regulatory colleges and so fall under the corresponding jurisdiction as well.

Both colleges have accreditation processes that oversee all active programs. Learners at this stage are represented by professional resident organizations that are established provincially.

Stage Four: Secondary Residency

After three years of primary residency, those learners involved in internal medicine or pediatrics then further segregate into about thirty subspecialties within these two disciplines. In addition, after two years, family medicine trainees have the option of undertaking a third year in an area of special interest, such as addiction medicine, care of the elderly, emergency medicine, enhanced surgical skills, anesthesia, obstetrics, palliative care, or sports medicine. Most family residency learners choose to undertake the third year and concentrate their practice in the focus area.

This stage is again influenced by both the College of Family Physicians and Royal College specialty committees. The Canadian matching service, which was active at the end of medical school, again plays a key role in coordinating and processing applications to the Royal College subspecialties. Accreditation agencies, hospital and clinical teaching sites, and provincially based professional resident organizations also exert considerable influence at this stage.

Stage Five: Tertiary Residency

As medical knowledge and therapeutic interventions have accelerated, many learners have chosen to undertake further training to develop specialized skills in these evolving fields. This is particularly true in many surgical disciplines as well as in several medical specialties, such as cardiology, gastroenterology, respirology, and neurology. These are informal training programs engaged by learners who individually contact specific clinical groups that are prepared to provide the training. These tend to be termed fellowships and have *ad hoc* funding arrangements. They may be funded by the teachers themselves who are supported in their clinical service delivery by the fellows. The fellows, who are now fully qualified in their subspecialty, may be working part time (colloquially called "moonlighting") to support themselves as they engage in this further training.

Stage Six: Qualification for Practice

At the end of training, learners must apply for a license to practice. This process is controlled by provincial and territorial regulators ("colleges" or "councils"), which, again, are independent in their determinations but do collaborate and share practices. General requirements include completion of a training program approved by the College of Family Physicians or Royal College and successful completion of Medical Council examinations. Both of these steps require a university medical degree. In addition, hospitals are independently responsible for allowing physicians to practice within their facilities, granting them so-called privileges, the scope of which varies based on specialty. This generally requires good standing with the provincial or territorial regulator and approval by the medical chief of staff who relies on specialty-based department heads to review and approve individual qualifications.

Putting It All Together

So, given all this background, let's return to a fundamental question: "Who's in Charge?" The following table attempts to list all the institutions, colleges, accrediting bodies, student and professional organizations, councils, committees, programs, and regulatory bodies that play a role somewhere along the way. Some of these are large and longstanding, such as universities and the Medical Council. Others are small, institutionally, or even departmentally, based bodies.

Regardless of age or size, all are highly successful in fulfilling their specific mandates. All those mandates are necessary to the education and qualification of physicians who will serve the Canadian public. But how did we evolve to become such a complex and segregated (dare we say "siloed") landscape? Not by primary intent, to be sure. Rather, all these entities arose to address emerging needs as medicine grew and became more specialized and complex. With expanding needs, new bodies were developed and empowered to take ownership for that particular issue, with highly capable people recruited to carry the torch.

Stage	Admissions	Primary Medical Education / Career Prep	Primary Residency	Sub-Specialization	Fellowship or Enhanced Skills	Qualification for Practice
Who's involved?	• 17 Medical Schools • Accrediting bodies • Numerous foreign medical schools	• Medical schools (17) • MCC • Regulators (13) • Accrediting Bodies • CaRMS • PG Training Programs (30) • Medical Student Societies (11) • Provincial and Territorial Ministries (13) • Interest Groups (?)	• Medical schools (17) • MCC • CCFP • Royal College Specialty Committees (30) • Accrediting Bodies • PG Training Programs (400) • Professional Resident Orgs (10) • Provincial and Territorial Ministries (13) • Hospitals (many...)	• CFPC • Royal College Specialty Committees (40) • Accrediting Bodies • PG Training Programs (150) • Professional Resident Orgs (10) • Provincial and Territorial Ministries (13) • Hospitals (?)	• Royal College AFC Committees (22) • Clinical Groups (ad hoc)	• Regulatory Colleges and Government Agencies (13)

However, and here's the rub, these entities are also functionally independent. Although there is much friendly collaboration and crosstalk, the fact remains that each is primarily dedicated to its own purpose and, it must be said, to protecting its own organizational integrity, place, and power in the process. The net effect is that, although any possible reform can be openly discussed, an invisible line exists at the point where any action threatens the core purpose or independence of the entities involved. Effectively, when it comes to reforms that require the cooperation of multiple players, everybody has a veto.

How Does This Work?

The Tokyo subway grid is illustrated below.

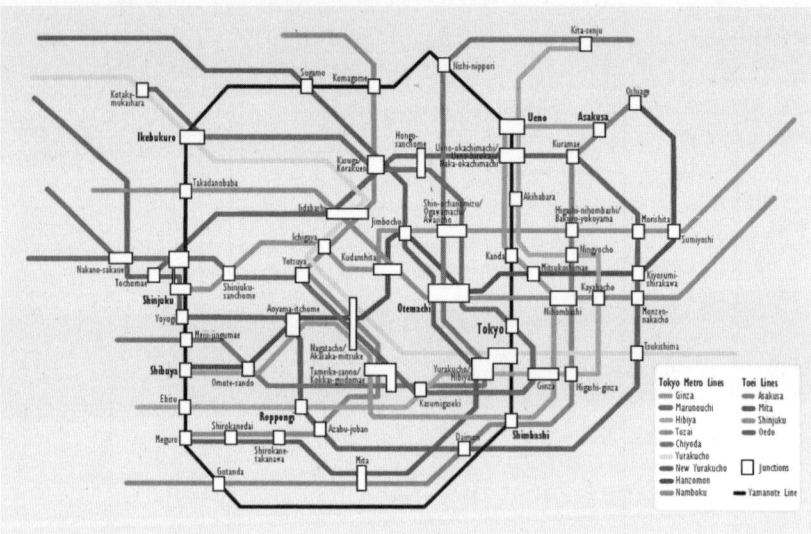

Retrieved from: https://commons.wikimedia.org/wiki/File:Tokyo_subway_map.PNG

It consists of hundreds of stations along multiple, interconnected lines. A passenger attempting to get from one point to another must travel through multiple stops. An obstruction at any station will stop the train and influence other interconnected lines. The system, I'm told, works exquisitely well despite its complexity, largely because someone oversees the whole grid in real time, and he or she is empowered to adjust or impose bypasses to keep the system running.

It doesn't hurt that they have people at each station pushing passengers onto packed trains.

System-level decision-making in the medical education process is similarly dependent on smooth passage through many independent bodies. However, there is no appropriately empowered higher-level oversight. Because everyone has a veto, and the exercise of those vetoes is based primarily on the specific institutional goals and preservation of each institution's position in the system, changes that threaten the authority of any one institution can be effectively stymied.

So…Who's in Charge?

Everybody, and nobody.

CHAPTER ELEVEN

Failing to Deliver

PREVIOUS CHAPTERS HAVE DESCRIBED THE impact felt by a steadily growing number of Canadians who are affected either directly or indirectly by the lack of community-based family physicians. We've also explored the impact on the physicians attempting to provide such care.

We've identified a number of changes occurred with respect to medical care that impact this problem. Specifically:

- Options for medical care and prevention of disease have grown dramatically. Conditions that were previously incurable are now quite treatable. All this has allowed for not only longer, but also much more active lives. Understandably, the expectations of Canadians of our medical profession have grown in parallel.
- Demographics and personal expectations of the medical profession are shifting dramatically too. Contemporary doctors strive to balance their commitment to work with their personal interests and health.

- Specialization results in a large number of disparate roles now encompassed by the qualification of the title "doctor."
- These roles vary not only in functions, but also with respect to the personal characteristics and interests of those taking them on. The medical community is, and needs to be, remarkably diverse in order to fill these roles.
- Providing comprehensive, continuing care in a generalist context is highly demanding, challenging, and underappreciated.
- The fee-for-service payment model most commonly used to compensate doctors is disadvantageous to family medicine practice.
- The admission process and traditional training paradigm provides a singular narrow gate through which trainees destined for all the diverse specialties must pass.
- Governance and oversight of the process for selecting and training doctors is shared among a large number of independent and well-established veto-enabled entities, making it difficult to achieve substantive system change.

These observations are neither mysterious nor malicious. They are natural developments that parallel the growth of medical care and social/political evolution of our society. They all contribute to, but none is individually responsible for, the deficiencies in medical care, which is the subject of this book. Solutions will need to be similarly multipronged. But before considering solutions, a key question must be posed. *How did we get here?* How is it we find ourselves with such a glaring inability to provide sufficient family doctors for the citizens of our country despite so many resources, organizational, and public attention to the problem? To approach that perplexing question, let's turn to first principles, as Aristotle might teach us, and consider how provision of services is *normally* controlled in our society.

The provision of a service or commodity is most directly driven by the demand for it—or at least it's supposed to be so.

Such relationship has been described as the concept of supply and demand. It can be traced back to ancient times and has been advanced by such prominent economic theorists as John Locke and Adam Smith. A phrase from the writings of James Denham-Steuart perhaps comes closest to encapsulating the concept in a manner that resonates with our contemporary medical dilemma:

> *"The nature of Demand is to encourage industry; and when it is regularly made, the effect of it is, that the supply for the most part is found to be in proportion to it..."*[17]

Basically, it postulates that the price for any product or service will be driven by a balance between how much is available from those able to supply it and how much it is desired (or required) by the consuming public. In essence, it describes a balance of interests between two parties—those who provide and those who consume (or require) that which is provided.

When in equilibrium, matching supply and demand provides a healthy balance of interests. Consumers are well provided for, and suppliers are under some competitive pressure to ensure quality and price control. The suppliers develop industries that employ folks who, in turn, become consumers who purchase various products. In short, everyone benefits. If there is an overabundance of any commodity, producers must drop prices to entice consumers. If there is an undersupply relative to needs (our current housing situation comes to mind as an example), costs tend to increase.

---

[17] Steuart, J. (1767). *An Inquiry into the Principles of Political Economy* (Book 2, Chapter 2), printed for A. Millar, and T. Cadell, in the Strand.

In fact, we go to great lengths to ensure that the balance is maintained. We have laws that prohibit monopolies so that no single provider can capture the market and become immune from competition. We have laws that prohibit collusion between suppliers. We do not allow price gouging during times of unexpectedly reduced supply, such as pandemics or natural disasters. In the case of products that we deem "essential," such as milk, we develop rigorous processes to regulate how many farms will be allowed to provide it, and even how much they will be allowed to supply, through quotas.

The undersupply of doctors in our society, which we've been exploring in the preceding chapters, would seem to be an instance where a dramatic and critical demand for an essential service has failed to trigger an adequate (or even close to adequate) increase in supply. Denham-Steuart's declaration that "*the nature of demand is to encourage industry*" has clearly not come to pass with respect to the "industry" of medical education, despite the clear, agitated, and sustained demands of the Canadian public. Why? What's gone wrong? Let's try to use this model to develop insights by examining both sides of that relationship.

What Drives "Demand"? What Do People Require of Their Doctors?

What do we need from the medical profession? Numerous studies have been undertaken asking the question, "What do patients want from their doctor?" There is much consistency and not much surprise in the responses, which range from pragmatic to humanistic considerations.

*People want their doctor to be **competent***. Although most patients can't fully assess their doctor's qualifications, they do get an intuitive sense through a physician's manner, ability to explain medical issues, and the way he or she proposes recommendations. They are willing to believe that their doctor's education and professional qualifications are all valid and in order. Over time, their trust is confirmed (or refuted) by the success or failure of the doctor's recommended treatments. To summarize, they want their doctors to be able to define and successfully resolve whatever difficulty they are experiencing at the moment. The primacy of this requirement increases with the urgency of the problem. In a pinch, simple competency may be all that matters.

*They wish their doctor to be **available** to them.* Most patients don't expect their doctor to be continuously at their beck and call and accept that they will have to engage emergency services when the need is urgent. However, they want to know how to access physician care and expect to be able to engage their doctor personally within a reasonable period of time.

*Patients would like to be able to access their doctor for **whatever problem** is troubling them.* Patients generally don't wish to self-diagnose or prioritize their concerns, nor should they be expected to. They do fully recognize that medical care has become complex and specialized and appreciate that no individual doctor will be able to manage whatever problem befalls them. However, they would like to have someone to whom they can turn with whatever is troubling them, to help sort out what is and isn't urgent, what can be resolved easily, and what requires further assessment and consultation. Even if that doctor isn't able to fully treat their problem, their interest and involvement in their ongoing care is very much desired and effective in ensuring the care is effectively provided, with accurate information about their condition handed off to each person who interacts with them.

*Patients want their doctor to **listen to them**.* Patients want to be heard. They know their doctor is busy and will see many other patients that day, but they expect to have the doctor's undivided attention for whatever time they are together, even if it just a few minutes.

*Patients **want to understand** what's wrong with them and what the plan is to get better.* Patients more and more wish to have some appreciation of their medical condition. Their doctor's effectiveness and simple willingness to help them understand the problem goes a long way to promoting trust and ensuring they engage and follow recommended treatments effectively.

*Patients want their doctor to **know them**.* They would like for the relationship to go beyond minimal medical facts and extend to some understanding of their particular life circumstances, challenges, and preferences. In fact, their confidence in their doctor's ability to diagnose and treat them will be enhanced if they believe those decisions are rooted in an understanding of those personal circumstances, such as a recent death in the immediate family or financial distress.

*Patients would like their doctors to be concerned not only with the treatment of active disease, but with its **prevention**.* Although this is by no means universal, a growing number of people are aware of and concerned about doing all they can to prevent getting ill and detecting illness as soon as possible in order to minimize its impact on themselves and their loved ones.

*Patients expect that their doctors to show **compassion**.* The word "compassion" comes up in almost every survey of patient preferences. Patients would like their doctor to go beyond the simple provision of service to care about them on a genuinely human, interpersonal level. They wish, to put it simply, a professionally personal relationship rather than a strictly provision-of-service, businesslike relationship.

Taking all of this into account and considering the wide variety of medical issues patients may encounter through their lives, it seems obvious they will require the services of multiple "types" of doctors through the course of their lives. The era of "one doctor for whatever ails you" is clearly a thing of the past. Patients have a steadily increasing need for doctors who are highly skilled in specific areas of medical care. They will need to be able to access such physicians as a new need arises and, hopefully, disengage as that need resolves. However, the need for *the one doctor* who will be a continuing presence in their lives, available for whatever ails them, interested in disease prevention and health maintenance, interested in them personally, and embodying the attributes listed, remains essential.

Public attention has recently and rightfully been centered on family medicine, which provides most of the comprehensive, continuing, preventive, personalized, compassionate care that patients seek. However, many other specialties experience similar challenges in meeting the demand for their services. Psychiatry, pediatrics, pathology, and oncology are prominent examples at this time.

In addition to the obvious impacts of a family doctor shortage on the simple provision of these medical services, the lack of sufficient physicians also robs patients of any choice they have in determining their care provider. Patients who, for whatever reason, are dissatisfied with their physicians have no alternative options available to them. Getting back to our supply–demand relationship, reduced demand has the effect of requiring suppliers to make their particular product more attractive, either through enhanced quality or reduced cost. In the context of massively excessive, unmet demand, there is no such motivation.

Bottom line: we need more doctors. Moreover, we need doctors who are trained and able to provide an increasing array of services.

It's also important to keep in mind that the supply issue is not because we lack sufficient young people who would like to become doctors. Each year, thousands of eager and capable young people fail to be accepted into Canadian medical schools despite much effort and preparation. Many thousands of young people travel to other countries and undertake great personal expense to study medicine. As noted earlier, it's widely considered that there are at least as many Canadians studying abroad as are studying at domestic medical schools. The bottleneck in the supply chain, quite clearly, is admission to medical school.

Why Has Our Obvious and Massive Demand for Doctors Not Resulted in Increased Supply?

1. Supply–demand disconnect
The first and most obvious reason is that supply–demand principles apply most clearly to an economic model in which the consumer pays for the product. In such systems, the supplier's income and viability are entirely dependent on the consumer, who can choose between competing providers. Our social model of universal and publicly funded health care is highly effective in ensuring everyone gets care for urgent problems regardless of their economic circumstances. The vast majority of Canadians (the author included) would not like to see that "safety net" compromised. However, there is no escaping the consequence that our funding model de-links demand from supply. In short, the supplier (medical education) is under no pressure to meet the demand (the public's need for doctors).

In fact, the current model very effectively *isolates* the consumer from the supplier. Health care consumers (patients) are unable to choose from product options or fully assess (or impact) the value of the product they are receiving. In such a de-linked system, the products (doctors) are free to choose how and to whom they will provide their services, with very little fear of criticism from patients who will feel grateful for whatever care they can secure.

As we've seen in previous chapters, university-based medical schools are the *de facto* entry point of the supply chain for the vast majority of doctors who practice in Canada. The physician workforce required to provide contemporary care has diversified and expanded as required by exploding medical knowledge and therapeutics. However, recruitment to the profession remains the domain of independent, university-based medical schools that admit undifferentiated students without reference to societal requirements regarding either the specialty or location of the products of the educational process. Moreover, the highly competitive admission process unintentionally selects for qualities at odds with those that would promote interest and success in family medicine. The funding of those schools, which comes largely from both government transfers and student tuitions, is not contingent on addressing contemporary societal needs. They therefore bear no direct responsibility for those problems and are not held to account by their funders, despite the fact that most of their funding comes from public sources and is thus provided by the very taxpayers whose needs are going unmet.

2. Economic disconnect

In addition, the model by which most doctors are compensated provides disproportionate incentives that are not aligned with public needs. As we saw in Chapter 7, the model favors procedural care over direct patient interactions, particularly ongoing repeat assessments, such as those required for the comprehensive, continuing, preventive care model.

3. Not allowing doctors to be doctors

To make matters even worse, the practice environment in which most family physicians function requires them to spend significant amounts of time with paperwork, correspondence, and advocating for their patients, rather than seeing, assessing, and treating patients. It also requires them to manage their work as small businesses—roles for which they are neither trained nor interested. And without the agility or ability to adjust prices or strategy. In other words, the system takes doctors away from core medical roles and renders them business managers with little power and insufficient training to manage.

Put another way, it wastes physician time with the consequence that individual doctors are able to see fewer patients.

In short, the economics of health care is not only delinking supply from demand, but also magnifying the dilemma we are struggling with.

4. Limited training capacity

A commonly cited issue is that training is long and expensive. Training more doctors, it's said, is something we simply can't afford. Universities and medical schools are already cash-strapped, and students are already emerging from their education with significant debt. As medical care has diversified and evolved, practice-relevant training has simply been added onto existing processes without reconsideration of ultimate needs and the overall educational pathway. The process of career selection and specialization occurs in parallel to active training. Consequently, medical education is a long, multifaceted process with multiple independently administered stages and embedded competitive application points. To make matters worse, medical schools are already experiencing great difficulties securing clinical learning settings for their students, particularly in areas such as family medicine, obstetrics, pediatrics, and psychiatry. The shortage of family doctors in our communities, of course, makes it even more difficult.

5. Change is difficult. Who's responsible and where to start?

As we've also seen in previous chapters, the medical education supply line is not a single process with clear oversight. It is, in fact, a series of sequential steps and processes, each governed by groups, institutions, and organizations with independent authority limited to their particular component. There is no unified locus of control, and no single entity bears responsibility for the central problem of inadequate supply.

What to Do? How Would a Healthy System Operate? Lessons from the Fast-Food World

Before 1948, the restaurant service was exclusively based on the model that required patrons to sit at tables and select from menus full of various options that were prepared on demand and served to them by waitresses or waiters who interacted with them and shuttled food from kitchen to table. We still enjoy this dining experience today but, back then, there was no other option.

But times were changing. More and more people had cars and wanted food options outside the home. They were interested in spending less time getting their meals, without sacrificing taste or quality. Two brothers who had been working in the motion picture industry as laborers and whose father had operated an early highway "food stand" recognized the changing needs and came up with a radical restaurant concept. It featured no tables and a menu that was centered on a single item—hamburgers—which could be prepared in large quantities very quickly and efficiently, such that they were ready to be served immediately on request. Patrons could order their meals at a counter and get them within a few minutes handed to them in (astonishingly, at the time) a paper bag! If they wished, they could even remain in their car, and someone would come out to take their order and deliver it to them a few minutes later. All this might seem quite obvious today but, at that time, Richard and Maurice McDonald were doing something completely novel and taking considerable risks. They opened their first McDonalds outlet in California that year and, as we know, revolutionized the food service industry.

What did they do? They examined changing needs and were willing to drastically depart from the tried and true. They were true innovators.

In his remarkable book *The Innovator's Dilemma*, the late Clayton Christensen describes *innovation* as a change in the "processes by which an organization transforms labor, capital, materials, and information into products and services of greater value." *Disruptive* innovations threaten previously accepted (and previously successful) management practices. In fact, they require a reconsideration of those historically successful principles and practices.

But hold on—is it reasonable to apply an organizational business model and lessons learned from a successful hamburger franchise to a complex, academically anchored and multifaceted process in which *multiple* organizations have independent roles? Is it reasonable to consider the education of doctors as a "product" comparable to photocopy machines or fast food?

Behind those two key questions lurks the answer to the "How did we get here?" conundrum. We're here because we have *not* accepted or engaged the problem as a failure to produce an adequate supply of doctors and there is no "organization" accountable for the problem.

And so, to take this discussion further, let's make a couple of theoretical assumptions. Let's assume there is an organization or responsible body of some type tasked with and given authority to address our doctor shortage. How would it get underway? How might its first meeting proceed? Surely, there would be a recognition of the need for true innovation.

Such innovation begins with examining a problem pragmatically and considering strategic solutions without the restrictions and conventions of current practice. Starting from scratch makes space for fresh and unhindered perspectives, from which unexpected approaches can emerge. They may not be easy to implement and are often seen as "disruptive," but they hold the promise of advancing the industry in ways not previously imagined.

If we accept that the key underlying issues are those "disconnects" listed earlier, a few such disruptive strategies emerge.

In the next chapters we will consider three such disruptive innovations that are intended to address the various key "disconnects" that our supply–demand analysis has exposed. They are chosen to address three potential points of intervention—*entry* to the profession, the *educational process* itself, and the *practice environment* family physicians will encounter. To be clear, these are not the only potential options but are chosen as key strategic opportunities to improve the supply of family physicians, which is so critical to the health of our patients and health care system.

CHAPTER TWELVE

Disruptive Innovation 1: Connecting Medical School Admissions to Societal Needs

IN CHAPTER 6, WE REVIEWED the current process for medical school admissions and drew several critical observations:

1. Almost all (98%) students accepted into medical school go on to become practicing physicians. There are very limited alternative routes to medical practice in Canada. Consequently, admission to medical school constitutes *de facto* admission to the medical profession.
2. There is no consistent or centralized approach. Decisions about the criteria used to assess applicants and process for their review are the independent domain of the seventeen (soon to be twenty) medical schools, which are almost all housed in universities and

entrusted to admissions committees, the membership and terms of reference of which are determined by university policy.
3. The criteria and processes used to assess medical school admissions are poorly aligned with the qualities and attitudes required of practicing physicians. This is particularly the case for generalist specialties such as family medicine.
4. The admission process imposes great demands and stresses on young applicants, which can be damaging to their personal development.
5. The admission process imposes significant barriers to many groups, particularly those from families without advanced education in previous generations, from smaller communities, and from less financially advantaged families.
6. The current process fails to account for the tremendous diversity of medical practice options and differences in qualities and skills required.
7. The current admission process is not linked or accountable to societal requirements for various specialties.

Given these considerations, it is hardly surprising that we are experiencing deficiencies of medical specialists, particularly family physicians who provide the vital primary, comprehensive, and continuing care that ensures the smooth functioning of the entire health care system. How can all this be addressed? Put another way, how would one construct an admission process if starting from scratch and recognizing the contemporary needs of our society for medical doctors of all specialties? A few suggestions:

Develop standards for admission that are relevant to modern medical practice
In determining the academic and non-academic criteria for admission, the requirements of medical *practice*, not of medical *school*,

should be the primary considerations. Medical school admission is not simply about entry to an area of academic interest, it is entry to a life's work. Applicants should be assessed relative to the requirements of that work, their understanding of the role, and their demonstrable commitment to it. This will require a complete back-to-basics approach, setting aside longstanding assumptions about the value of (clearly unreliable) grades and test results. Some items to consider in a refreshed approach might include:

- commitment to service,
- ability to engage and relate to people, including diverse populations,
- ability to deal with uncertainty,
- adaptability in the face of change,
- problem solving,
- resilience,
- teamwork.

In addition, the admission process should consider the question of how such attributes could best be identified, actively seeking objective evidence, particularly lived experiences that demonstrate applicants have met these criteria. This means going beyond simple applicant testimonials and honed interview skills. The process should put a premium on lived experience and mitigate the phenomenon of application engineering.

Develop different approaches for the recruitment of different types of doctors

Admission processes must recognize the diversity of medical practice specialties now required and provide more targeted and specialty-specific approaches. Modern medical care requires all specialties and likely more in the future, but they don't all require the same interests, strengths, and aptitudes among all those who practice. The admission process must reflect this diversity. The concept of a single port of entry to so many diverse but vital practice options is a vestige of the past and simply no longer reasonable or viable. The notion that we need to devote time in medical school to career exploration has some merit, but it is also entirely reasonable to expect that young people considering a career in medicine will have based that decision on some realistic exploration, prior to admission, of the life's work they are hoping to undertake. Even if limited to general fields of practice such as family medicine, medical and surgical specialties, mental health, and laboratory medicine, such pre-admission streaming could greatly facilitate a more targeted admission process and lessen the considerable pressure medical programs now face to devote time and attention to assisting students through that process after entry.

Expand the admission process to attract and welcome individuals who have had some personal experience in other fields of health care

Prior life experience in professions such as nursing, lab technology, and rehabilitation therapy provides maturity and a realistic understanding of the scope and role of medicine. Because of the various barriers to medical education described in Chapter 6, many highly capable individuals may have never considered themselves viable applicants given the current competitive process for medical school but have the potential to make tremendous contributions as community-based physicians if given the opportunity. Their personal experiences and pre-existing bonds within communities of practice make it much more likely that they will return to those communities and become long-term contributors. The admission process should be open to such applications.

Be honest and forthright with applicants about the realities of a medical career and what it is not

A career in medicine can be, without question, immensely rewarding and satisfying. Doctors have the capacity to positively impact the lives of the individual patients they encounter and the communities in which they live. They are well remunerated, secure, and highly regarded. However, their profession is also very demanding from entry to retirement. It is, essentially, a life of service to others where expectations are high, errors can have catastrophic results, and personal accolades are few and far between. We need to dramatically alter our pre-medical school messaging. A medical education is not a prize to be sought after nor a reward for scoring perfect grades. It should be a means to an end—that end being a deep desire to improve the lives of those unknown and unfiltered "others" among us in need of care and assistance.

Potential applicants should have that desire. They also deserve to be realistically informed about the nature of the career they are considering. Of all medical specialties, family medicine is the most complete in terms of its ability to provide that comprehensive and continuing care to patients. If all admitted students were fully prepared for the realities of medical practice and if our admission process was effective in identifying truly service- and patient-oriented individuals, it would be the natural choice of most students. Family medicine is a high and noble calling.

Be willing to say, "This isn't working out."

Is an almost zero percent attrition rate from medical school a sign of admission success or a failure to guide and support career development? Despite best practices and good intentions on the part of all involved, there will inevitably be instances where an individual admitted to medical school is unsuited, uncomfortable, or simply unhappy with the career they've chosen. Currently, medical schools feel compelled to ensure every student eventually graduates, and failure to do so is seen as an indictment of their ability to provide personal support and educate effectively. Students, having successfully navigated the highly competitive admission process, are under tremendous personal, family, financial, and societal pressure to complete what they have begun. They can feel trapped in a career which they now realize is much different than what they imagined. Failure to address this dilemma can lead to long-term dissatisfaction, only to have devastating consequences for these individuals, their families, and their eventual patients. In short, failing to identify and address these admission "mismatches" is a disservice to all involved, particularly the student. Generally, this "mismatch" is related to discomfort with the intensity of interpersonal interactions required and personal and emotional commitment that goes with it. Feeling unable to escape, they will opt for a role within medical practice in which they will feel most comfortable, which usually involves very predictable roles with limited personal interactions. Family medicine would be far down that list.

Develop approaches that will overcome the social and financial barriers

Doing so will increase access to medical school for a wider range of people, including those who have already had some experience in other health care professions. In addition to being intrinsically fairer and providing a more diverse physician workforce, this will certainly result in more people with experiences and backgrounds in keeping with comprehensive, continuing care in smaller communities. There are many obvious options to consider, including:

- Inviting more applications from people who have already had some experience in the health care workforce (as above).
- The elimination of admission expenses of dubious value such as the MCAT.

- De-emphasizing volunteerism unavailable to financially disadvantaged applicants.
- Enhanced and appropriately targeted scholarship opportunities.
- Developing cooperative training programs with an embedded (and paid) work placement.
- Providing clinical placements that not only develop skills and promote professional development, but also provide income.

Link admissions to societal needs
Finally, and perhaps most importantly, the medical school admission process must recognize and address its primary responsibility to address the needs of the society that supports it through public funding and is critically dependent upon it to meet the health care needs of all citizens. The long training time involved in preparing students for practice makes it difficult to rapidly adjust to changing needs, but careful analysis of prospective workforce requirements in various specialties, while considering the number, age, and practice locations of current practitioners, is available and could be used to guide recruitment. As our current crisis in the medical workforce so well illustrates, this is not an academic but rather a public policy issue. Medical education, after all, is largely supported through public funding. Although students pay tuitions, these cover only about one third of the costs of their education, and postgraduate students (residents) are fully paid with funds provided by provincial governments. Is it all unreasonable to expect a greater degree of accountability to the evolving needs of those bearing the costs?

Unify the admission process
This selection process is simply too important and vital to the public interest to be entrusted to so many disparate, independent, internally accountable, and continually renewing committees. Ideally, there should be a single process by which applications are received and assessed and successful applicants are assigned to various schools

across the country. At the very least, consistent standards and processes must be established that govern the objectives and processes for medical school admission.

All this, it must be acknowledged, flies in the face of longstanding tradition and established practice. Change of this magnitude will threaten the autonomy of venerable institutions that have struggled honestly and valiantly to provide valuable service and preserve their role in the process. But broader views are required to address the physician workforce crisis that is upon us, and reconsideration of the entry point to practice is a necessary step toward effective change. On the positive side, changes will likely be welcome by many beleaguered admission groups that are attempting to deal individually with mounting pressures to meet increasing concerns in isolation.

CHAPTER THIRTEEN

Disruptive Innovation 2: Connecting Medical Education to Societal Needs

HAVING SELECTED STUDENTS WHO ARE committed to careers in community-based family medicine, how do we best prepare them for their career?

As outlined previously, the current training process has several shortcomings.

The requirement for undifferentiated students to explore career options and engage in competitive selection processes distracts from and diminishes educational goals. It can also give rise to an inherent conflict between the goals of the program and learners. Medical education programs are primarily intended to provide undifferentiated, "pluripotential" learning. In biology, the term "pluripotential" describes cells that have the potential to give rise to several different specialized cell types. Learners are increasingly focused on exploring specific career tracts and may see much of the training irrelevant to their purpose, and even in conflict with their desire to "match" to a desired training program.

The "handover" of learners between educational programs and institutions (particularly from university-based undergraduate medical education to employment-based residencies) also gives rise to inefficiencies and thereby hampers coordinated, integrated learning. It also contributes to a progressive accumulation of debt by tuition-paying undergraduate students, even though they participate actively in care delivery for at least part of that time.

In the case of family medicine in particular, several additional issues are relevant.

- Medical education is institutionally, and largely, hospital-based, whereas family medicine is largely practiced in the community. Students therefore have limited exposure to authentic practice settings.
- Medical education is conducted largely along specialty lines with the result that, in a curriculum endeavoring to provide exposure to all specialties, students will be exposed largely to non-family medicine specialists.
- The medical education process, structured along specialty lines, gives the impression that family medicine is the beginning of understanding of disease processes, with the implication that only more differentiated specialists provide fully evolved patient care.
- For most of the students who survive the current admission process, therapeutics seem inherently more exciting and cutting-edge than holistic diagnostics, further adding to the impression that the generalist is less critical to care than the more highly differentiated specialist.

All this results in students receiving a distorted impression of the role and importance of family medicine, which no doubt influences career selection.

To make matters worse, our current model of early medical education is inherently inefficient and wasteful of a key resource—specifically, patients who are willing to be seen and examined by students, thus providing learning opportunities without much, or any, enhancement of the care they're receiving. As we've seen in previous chapters, the current process is based on acceptance of an individual who is uncommitted to any particular discipline and therefore spends considerable time and clinical learning placements ensuring students get exposure to all disciplines and specialties in order to make that determination. Medical schools go to great lengths to ensure all students are involved in a wide variety of patient encounters and experiences, including surgeries, labor and delivery, gynecologic assessments, pediatric assessments, and psychiatric assessments. This is despite the fact that most of those students will never provide those services in practice, and those who do will get that definitive training in the context of their specialty training. They also spend considerable curricular time invested in the career differentiation and application process—all of which consumes scarce dollars and teaching time. If the process were shorter and if students only undertook training that was relevant to their eventual practice setting, there would be less demand for clinical placements and costs would be considerably less. In addition, practicing physicians would be much more likely to engage students participating in their practices if they knew those students would eventually be taking up positions as their colleagues and perhaps even practice partners.

And so, what to do? If one were able to start from the beginning, how would they structure the ideal family medicine educational process?

- That program would be designed and structured to prepare learners specifically for that career.
- It would have the goal of graduating practice-ready practitioners without the need of movement between different institutional governance bodies, each with different rules.
- It would have embedded community-based experiences that replicate practice and prepare students appropriately.
- It would allow students to engage in roles within community-based clinical practice that reflected their evolving knowledge, skills, and scope of practice.
- Training would be carried out in settings where effective team-based, multi-professional practice was available.
- Family physicians would be involved and visible in all aspects of the educational process. Other specialists involved would understand the needs of family medicine and the value of effective collaborative care. Family physicians would be working side by side with other specialists on the main stage, not relegated to the backstage.
- Learners would not transition suddenly from being tuition-paying students to salary-earning residents but, rather, be compensated for clinical placements as these placements arose in the course of their training. As their roles in the clinical environment became more prominent, the balance between tuition paid and salary earned would evolve in parallel.
- There would be a single and common institutional governance overseeing all aspects of the training program, including admissions, curriculum, community teaching sites, and faculty engagement.
- And, most importantly, it would begin by admitting people already committed to careers in community-based family medicine. There would be no need for further distracting career exploration or competitive admission processes.

Readers not familiar with medical education may be wondering at this point, "So if that makes sense, why not just go ahead? In fact, why aren't you already doing it that way?"

For an answer to that excellent question, we must return to the Tokyo subway analogy of Chapter 10. Medical education is a journey with many stations along the way, each with its own requirements for admission and complex transfers along the way. Each of them is overseen by multiple institutions, organizations, colleges, agencies, and committees, all of which would need to be aligned and willing to relinquish some component of their individual authority and autonomy. In short, no one's driving the train and very few are focused on the ultimate outcome, which should be to provide doctors trained to meet societal needs.

CHAPTER FOURTEEN

Is Disruptive Innovation Realistic Within Medical Education?

AS WE REVIEWED IN CHAPTER 10, there are many independent institutions, professional colleges, and political bodies involved in the process of selecting and training physicians. In the absence of any point of central control, how can the sort of major reform that's required be achieved? Fortunately, there is a critical lever that has not yet been fully engaged.

All the President's Men is a 1976 drama that depicts the process of uncovering the Watergate scandal. In this hit film, the anonymous informant known as "Deep Throat" urges the investigating reporters to "follow the money." By doing so, they were able to isolate the source of corruption by tracing the financial trail of the individuals involved.

As we've reviewed, the selection and education of doctors are controlled by universities, professional colleges, residency programs, and councils. All of these have one important thing in common. If we "follow the money," we'll find that the majority of their funding emanates from provincial governments. These public dollars support all aspects of physician education. Provincial governments are ultimately responsible for ensuring these dollars are used to address the needs of the people they represent. Would it not be reasonable (in fact, expected) that the funding comes with some expectation that selection and programming are coordinated and driven by societal requirements for the appropriate number and type of physicians trained? In practical terms, this would involve measuring and holding medical schools accountable for the quality of their outputs (i.e., the doctors they graduate) rather than focusing on high undergraduate GPAs and MCAT scores of the students they admit.

At the end of the day, the buck stops (and starts) with our provincial governments and ministries. They, and they alone, hold the lever to meaningful reform. If, for example, the funding of 25 percent of medical school positions were sequestered for students committed to careers in community-based family medicine and programming to specifically prepare them for such careers, medical schools would be required to develop such admission processes and curricula very quickly indeed. Is it possible? Within a year of its approval, Queen's University was able to develop just such processes for a subgroup of its medical class at a satellite campus located in Durham Region. These students, selected based on their interest and aptitude for careers in community-based family medicine, began a six-year program to provide targeted, community-integrated training in September 2023.[18]

Yes, it can be done.

---

[18] Sanfilippo, A. J., & Philpott, J. (2023, October 1). Family doctor shortage: Medical education can help address critical gaps, starting with a specialized program. *The Conversation*.

CHAPTER FIFTEEN

Disruptive Innovation 3: Restructure Care Delivery to Better Meet Patient and Physician Needs

EVERY DAY, AT EVERY HOSPITAL across Canada, patients make their way to emergency departments with non-urgent medical problems.

Some have pain that they've never experienced before and isn't getting better.

Some have complex medical problems that have been chronic and predictable but are now spiraling out of control for no apparent reason.

Some have been ill for several days with an illness that they still think is "just a cold or flu" but isn't improving. In fact, it's getting worse.

Some have fallen and may have injured themselves.

Some, brought in by concerned neighbors or family members, are getting confused and simply not managing well at home.

These folks, and many, many others, don't have problems that they or anyone would consider truly urgent. They know this. They know how overcrowded and stressed the emergency departments have become. They don't want to be there.

But they have nowhere else to go.

In the health system in which they live (and most Canadians believe it to be one of the best in world assuring all of "universal" access), for anyone without a family doctor, or seeking care after standard office hours, the emergency department is the only option available.

We've also learned that many qualified family doctors, like Rachel from Chapter 2, are abandoning comprehensive care. The settings they worked in did not allow them to deliver what they considered optimal care, nor did they provide a satisfying or rewarding work environment.

What's going on? To examine this further, let's take a closer look at how this is all playing out in real life with actual patients.

Sylvia's Story

Sylvia works as a sales representative in a large department store. She lives alone and considers herself fortunate to have a family doctor. For about a month, she's been waking up at night with a burning sensation in the middle of her abdomen, just below her ribcage. It seems to get better if she sits up and, on the advice of a friend, she's been taking antacid tablets, which seems to help. She's tried sleeping in different positions and avoiding food after suppertime, but the problem is persistent and has started disturbing her sleep.

She realizes the problem doesn't really constitute an emergency, and so she calls her family doctor's office to make an appointment to be seen. After several attempts and a number of questions from the person taking her call, she succeeds in getting an appointment scheduled for three weeks out.

During these three weeks, the problem worsens, with increasing severity and duration of pain, which has lingered into the morning and is no longer responsive to the antacid tablets. She's getting progressively weaker and more fatigued from the lack of sleep.

The appointment takes place in the doctor's office, which is shared with several other family physicians. Sylvia drives herself to the appointment, pays for a half day of parking, and makes her way to the crowded waiting room, where she lines up to see the receptionist to "report in." She waits about 20 minutes and is finally called into an examining room where she's told the doctor will be in shortly.

Now let's examine the possibilities that might arise as a result of the doctor's assessment:

1. The doctor may conclude that there's a clear and treatable cause for Sylvia's problem, prescribe some remedy, and arrange for a follow-up call or appointment to ensure things are getting better.
2. The doctor may not be sure about the cause of the pain but feel the situation is not urgent, thus recommending some tests to investigate. The tests will be scheduled, each independently and likely at different locations. Sylvia will be given appointments for these tests and then a re-appointment with the family doctor to review the results. All this will require several appointments that Sylvia will have to make, but all the while missing work, which will take several weeks. These tests, once complete, will need to be interpreted by another doctor with appropriate expertise, who will then generate a report that will, eventually, find its way to Sylvia's doctor with findings and recommendations.
3. The doctor may decide that Sylvia requires the services of a dietician or therapist. In that case, such appointments will need to be

scheduled and attended. Subsequently, the doctor will follow up with Sylvia to assess her progress.

4. The doctor may feel that a consultation is required with a specialist in stomach disorders (a gastroenterologist) or possibly a surgeon. The doctor will request that appointment, and Sylvia will be told to go home to await a call and appointment time, which is anticipated to be at least a month and will likely lead to a need for further testing.
5. The doctor may feel Sylvia's situation is concerning enough to require urgent attention and direct Sylvia to go to the emergency department of the local hospital. The doctor may call that department and speak to the physician there to share the details of Sylvia's problem and her concerns, to hopefully expedite Sylvia's assessment.

Where Family Medicine Is Practiced

A generation ago, family doctors practiced in many settings within their community and encountered their patients in many ways outside the office setting, including:

- Arranging to meet patients in the local emergency department.
- Admitting and caring for their patients in local hospitals.
- Visiting their patients who were in the hospital.
- Visiting patients at long-term care and chronic care facilities.
- Visiting patients in their home.

Family doctors were ubiquitous and welcome in all these settings, the choice of which was determined by the needs of the patient.

Obviously, much has changed. Most family medicine and primary care (particularly in larger centers) is carried out in office settings. More and more, patients must find their way to their doctors, whose scope of activity has become much more limited to their offices or clinics. There are many entirely valid reasons for this dramatic change in the practice of family medicine. However, Sylvia's experience illustrates the shortcomings of office-based encounters. Of the potential outcomes of Sylvia's visit, only one could be fully addressed within that setting. A single doctor in an office encountering a patient with even a moderately complex or undifferentiated problem will likely not be able to resolve that problem at that visit. Simply put, the practice environment is often inadequate for the purpose.

The Consequences

Waiting to have a persisting and undefined medical problem resolved both prolongs suffering and causes stress, which can be debilitating. There is also an economic impact as patients struggle to juggle work schedules and get to appointments.

Depending on the ultimate cause of Sylvia's problem, the waiting time involved may be unsafe. As she waits longer and longer for a resolution, she may be not only suffering with pain, fatigue, and stress, but also at risk as the underlying problem remains active and potentially worsens.

The doctors involved are also impacted by this inadequate practice environment. Family doctors are trained to diagnose and treat a wide range of medical problems. However, to do so, they require access to diagnostic and therapeutic resources, much of which will not be available in an office setting. The increasing complexity of medical care has only amplified this gap. All this can lead to feelings of frustration and futility, which are powerful contributors to the problem of burnout.

In addition, this process adds considerably to the paperwork issue, which, as we've learned in previous chapters, has become a major source of inefficiency and dissatisfaction for family doctors.

- Every test that Sylvia's doctor orders requires a separate requisition to be completed, some of which require details of the patient's history and medications. They may also require blood work or other preliminary assessments that have to be carried out before the test can be completed.
- Every consultation requires a written request to the consulting physician, outlining the patient's background and reason for the referral.
- Every test that comes back must be read and results followed up. Abnormal test results must be addressed. In addition, advanced imaging tests like CT scans or MRI scans may uncover unsuspected findings that will require further evaluation and discussion with the patient.
- Finally, consultations usually come with recommendations for treatment or further investigation, which, again, often falls to the referring family doctor to address.

Because so many of the problems coming into an office-based practice can't be fully resolved in that setting, the office-based family doctor is dealing with an avalanche of information that is continually coming in and requires careful attention if patients are to receive appropriate care. For what technologists call a "single source of truth" to house all the continually changing data about any patient interacting with so many providers, the family doctor will need (and this assumes the electronic medical record functions) to review updates on patients at a torrid pace.

As discussed earlier, some of the changes doctors have adopted to cope with increasing demands in their work environment have had damaging effects.

Documenting information on computers during patient visits, though intended to improve efficiency, can be stressful to patients and erode trust.

The "one problem per visit" policy runs the real risk of increasing the downstream burden of care by deferring important issues that may persist or worsen and therefore require more visits and more resources. It can also artificially over-simplify complex patient problems and underestimate true system needs, thus depriving our medical system of comprehensive data about the diversity of concerns patients are in fact experiencing. Such information could inform the appropriate number and mix of specialists needed to meet societal needs. Guided by valid information, medical schools could adjust their focus as needed and government payers could incentivize them to allocate for these specialist spots accordingly.

It's easy to imagine that all this is economically inefficient, consumes valuable physician time, and leads to much frustration as well as physical and emotional fatigue. Multiple, disjointed tests and consultations carried out at different locations and at different times therefore have a financial as well as human cost that could be mitigated by bringing services and people together in an integrated fashion.

So, Can We Do Better?

Can we imagine a model of care delivery that would address the important needs of these patients who are reluctantly seeking non-urgent care in emergency departments and provide a more welcoming and effective practice environment for the Rachels of the world?

Yes. To meet the patient care needs, the model would need to meet some key criteria:

1. **Accessibility**. Patients would be able to review their concerns, and the doctor would attend to them without prolonged delays or complicated processes for establishing appointment times. As a first step, patients would be able to contact their doctor

(or a practice partner) by phone or virtual visit to discuss their concerns and best course of action, which might involve an expedited personal visit or any of the options described above for Sylvia. In addition to streamlining the process, this would reduce patient stress and ensure potentially serious concerns are addressed early on.
2. **Staffing** to meet a variety of needs. This would involve a team of professionals with a variety of knowledge and skills, capable of working together to provide services needed to patients who would likely have multiple problems or medical issues complicated by difficult personal circumstances.
3. **Connectivity** to diagnostics, urgent care, and a variety of specialty services that could be accessed smoothly and without delay.

To address the concerns expressed by many family physicians, the model would have to provide:

1. Freedom from (or at least support for) administrative and business management responsibilities.
2. Freedom from (or at least support for) clerical tasks such as note-taking and filling out forms. The mantra would be "Let the doctors be doctors."
3. A collegial, team environment where patient care and call responsibilities can be shared.
4. A work arrangement with built-in options that allow taking time off for vacation, professional development, or personal purposes.
5. The ability to combine the comprehensive care of their patients with an area of focused care or expertise which they're able to provide in parallel.
6. Easily accessible and effective support from specialists in key areas relevant to their patient population.

There is an adage worth borrowing from the world of anatomy that "form follows function." It basically means that structures that we develop, like those that evolve naturally, should be products of the function they are intended to provide. The converse is that developing a structure initially and expecting it to provide all the functions required will always have shortcomings.

In our case, the *form* that emerges from the *functions* we've described might be described as an "integrated care center" that provides both primary and intermediate (complex but non-urgent) level care in a multi-professional, well-managed, easily accessible center with seamless connections to diagnostics, consultation, and more acute care as required.

It would consist of a group of family physicians and affiliated health professionals who share similar goals and perspectives about their clinical roles, commitment to community service, and willingness to work in a more integrated model that prioritizes their primary role as physicians and other care providers.

Physicians are compensated at a negotiated annual rate, subject to reassessment every few years. Their package includes benefits for certain items and an optional pension arrangement.

A business manager (likely someone with an MBA and/or managerial experience) works with the physician group and is involved with decisions regarding what other allied health (e.g., nurses, therapists, dieticians) and administrative personnel are to be hired. The manager deals with all aspects of budgeting, human resources, and office management, which are derived from the principles and role descriptions developed and accepted by the physician group.

Physician staffing is developed based on preset assumptions regarding individual vacation time, conference leave, and scheduled sabbaticals for professional upgrading or personal reasons (such as maternity or paternity leaves). In other words, absences are built in and anticipated in the staffing model—in much the same way many small businesses in other industries plan well in advance for backfilling key personnel or hiring fractional staff or specialists as needed. Any business in any industry is not sustainable if it is "single-threaded"—otherwise, the organization's productivity sputters or screeches to a halt if a key person is missing. Right now, the vast majority of family practices in Canada are "single-threaded." We need to fix this.

The integrated care center, under this new model, is responsible for the care of a predetermined, geographically defined population within the community. People living in, or moving into, that community (or region) would be automatically registered with that center, in much the same way that they access schools or police and fire protection.

The expectations for this population are not based on the number of encounters or individual items of service, but rather on a series of outcome parameters that are defined in advance and intended to reflect more holistic care and outcomes. For example, the following items could be tracked on a semi-annual basis and compared to both preset targets and the same metrics for other similar organizations:

- Average time for a patient encounter with a physician (which could begin with a virtual encounter and lead to an in-person visit as needed).
- Number of patients reporting to emergency departments not requiring urgent care or admission.
- Prevalence of key preventable health issues, such as stroke, heart attacks, invasive skin cancers, bowel cancer, and lung cancer.
- Patient satisfaction with care to be determined through a confidential and randomly distributed survey.

Importantly, how those outcomes are achieved would be entirely at the discretion of the team. Unlike in the prior model, they would set a strategy just like an automobile company and design the performance indicators to fulfill the strategy. Their funding is not based on what specific things they do or organizational structures they develop, but rather based entirely on outcomes they achieve. The doctors are therefore free to be doctors and to use their training and ingenuity to engage in whatever methods they chose or to develop novel and innovative approaches.

They could, for example, choose to develop a completely virtual interface wherein one member of the team screens patient requests and determines a course of action for each, including the need for in-person assessments and how soon they need to schedule.

They could develop a culture whereby patients have an identified primary physician but also understand that they will encounter and get to know other members of the team who will be intermittently involved in their care.

In such a system, it would quickly become clear that engaging physicians in clerical tasks such as typing appointment summaries, completing forms, filling prescriptions, and submitting test requisitions is an inefficient and wasteful use of their time. With appropriate training and supervision, administrative support staff could be trained to perform such duties, freeing up physicians for patient encounters, counseling, and decision-making.

The team could choose to develop contractual relationships with other key specialists, such as internists, cardiologists, surgeons, obstetrician/gynecologists, psychiatrists, and pediatricians who would be available to the team to consult on individual patient issues. These contracted consultants would also coordinate appropriate responses by acting as liaisons to other specialists, diagnostics, or hospital-based services. Such arrangements would foster effective and collegial inter-professional collaborations with the engaged specialists. Being engaged as such a consultant would be at the discretion of the team and, within the broader community, be seen as a recognition of excellence and an expression of esteem.

From a societal and public health perspective, this arrangement would have fixed and understood costs in exchange for defined and agreed-to benefits. There is no need for unbendable definitions, accounting strictures, and negotiation terms on every potential item of service. The only relevant outcomes are those that are connected to a predefined strategy: they are truly important, agreed to in advance, and comparatively easy to track.

This is one model provided to illustrate a potential approach, but similar principles can be applied to variations as community needs evolve and physician preferences vary. It's also a model that can accommodate varying areas of focused interest among the participating physicians. A participating doctor with special interest in infectious diseases and public health, for example, could gain enhanced training in that discipline and become the group lead for such issues.

It's also interesting to consider what sort of physician would be attracted to such a practice arrangement. These would be people who are not only attracted to family medicine as a discipline, but also focused on patient outcomes, alleviating disease burden in general, developing innovative models of care delivery, being adept at thinking outside the box, and importantly, exhibiting a strong preference for working as part of a mutually supportive team.

But is this practical? Is it even possible given the resource constraints the provinces are already experiencing? Would it not make more sense to simply shovel money into more emergency departments, or more chronic care beds, to ease the burden on our acute care hospitals?

The answers to these valid questions should have two dimensions:

1. Does the proposed model provide better patient care and outcomes?
2. What are the resource implications?

The first question should be judged against the sort of outcome issues listed above. The resource issue must consider all collateral as well as direct expenses and savings. In other words, it's not just about what costs are incurred, but about what costs are reduced or avoided. Such comprehensive modeling must encompass the value of physician and nursing time and determine in which tasks it is best spent.

All this is to say that such options should be thoughtfully considered. Our patients need somewhere to turn for non-urgent issues, and family physicians need a practice environment that truly values and honors their skills and rewards them with personal satisfaction. Solutions to both issues may be one and the same.

CHAPTER SIXTEEN

Can We Change?

JEREMY HAS JUST FINISHED A grueling day and is finally leaving the hospital. Glancing at his watch and adding up expected travel times, he estimates that he'll reach home just in time to take his young daughter to her hockey practice, as he promised when he put her to bed last evening.

Jeremy graduated from medical school just last year and is in the first year of his family medicine residency. He's currently doing a six-week rotation on a general surgery service. His days are very full, assessing patients in the emergency department, admitting many to the hospital, ensuring they're prepared for their surgeries, assisting in the operating room, and caring for them as they recover. Today has been particularly hectic, but he's gotten through his long list of tasks and signed out to the resident on call. As he exits the hospital and approaches the parking lot, he feels comfortable that he's done everything expected of him. Good to go.

Then, he remembers Mrs. D'Souza and stops in his tracks.

Mrs. D'Souza is an 84-year-old lady he admitted a few days ago from the emergency department. She's a widow who lives alone.

Her children keep her in close contact but live in cities many hours away. She came to the hospital because of abdominal pain and has been found to have a tumor that is obstructing her colon and requires surgical excision—a hemicolectomy. She has some cardiac problems and diabetes, so this will not be a simple undertaking. In fact, it's quite risky, but there's really no other option given the obstruction.

Jeremy has been managing her investigations since admission, keeping her and her family informed along the way. Her English is limited, and so he's had to take extra time to explain things and understand her questions. They have "bonded." She sees him as "her doctor." She has come to look forward to his visits and trusts his guidance.

That morning, he visited her on rounds together with the chief surgeon and a team of more senior residents. The surgeon explained what they intended to do, outlined the risks, and asked whether she had questions or concerns. She agreed to the surgery, but Jeremy could see that she didn't fully understand everything that was said. She also seemed afraid and a little intimidated, such that she was unwilling to ask further questions. So, he stayed back, took her hand, and told her he would be back after rounds to speak with her further. She seemed very relieved.

Except he didn't. His day got very busy, and he forgot. Until now.

So, what to do? If he keeps his promise to Mrs. D'Souza, he will disappoint his daughter, again.

Jeremy's personal dilemma as he stands at the entrance of the hospital will be familiar to many. It also has some parallels to the situation we collectively find ourselves facing as we consider how, or even whether, to confront and resolve the family medicine crisis.

We have done what is expected of us, both individually and as collectives engaged in the education and support of physicians. No individual or institution bears singular responsibility for this crisis, nor are we individually empowered to bring about the substantial reforms that will be required.

Doing so will require everyone involved to step away from the processes and organizational structures that have, over long periods of time, been successful, seemingly reliable, and comfortable. It will also require trust that others involved in the process will make similar commitments. We will need some confidence that these others involved will match our willingness to engage in reform. It will, in short, require a leap of faith.

So, why change? Why risk what's working, even if imperfectly? After all, these days just maintaining the status quo, to prevent the ship from running aground, can seem like a victory.

The suggestions outlined in previous chapters, and others that will surely come forward from more creative sources, will be difficult and disruptive. In the end, as for Jeremy, there's only one reason to do so—because it's in the best interests of our patients and fellow citizens. As was introduced in Chapter 1, and as is apparent to all of us, they are suffering. They deserve better, and collectively, we can do better.

And so, like Jeremy standing at the hospital entrance, we must make a choice.

What will it be?

ACKNOWLEDGEMENTS

IF EVER THERE WAS A labor of love, this is it. But, as I've come to learn, love alone doesn't get a book published. It requires much advice, encouragement, shared wisdom, and practical guidance. In the case of this particular book, it's required all those things from two separate and rather disparate worlds: one that I knew very well; the other, not at all.

In exploring the shortcomings of medical education that underlie our current physician crisis, I was able to draw on several decades of immersion in these processes as a practicing physician, teacher, and educational lead.

It gave me an opportunity to hear from patients (always a doctor's best teachers) who were willing to share their personal stories and the impact of seeking care in an increasingly complex, fragmented, and intimidating network of people and services.

I was able to hear from educators and leaders involved in all aspects of the long and winding path from medical school admission to practice readiness.

I heard from many thoughtful and insightful students I'd encountered over the years. I heard of the excruciating admission experience and witnessed its effects. I also heard from medical school faculty members who developed and worked prodigiously to make that experience as fair and effective as possible.

I heard from students and residents about their struggle to find their way among the many medical specialty paths while learning everything they needed to learn to graduate and qualify.

I heard from practicing family physicians, many of whom I had known for years, and very graciously responded to requests for a conversation. All were very willing to candidly share their challenges, struggles, and disappointments.

I am particularly indebted to the many (over fifty at last count) undergraduate medical education deans who I had the opportunity to work with and get to know over my fifteen years in that role. Their dedication to maintaining the integrity of the educational process and willingness to share struggles and successes were continually inspiring and energizing. Many of the thoughts and insights contained in this book arose from these free-flowing discussions. I want to particularly acknowledge Drs. Bruce Wright, Beth Cummings, Melissa Forgie, Jay Rosenfield, and Gary Tithecott, who have become continuing sources of counsel and friendship.

Anyone with controversial and radical views benefits from the advice and guidance of folks whom they have known long enough and well enough to be trusted to tell the unvarnished truth. I am fortunate enough to have four such friends who, on any Sunday morning over cream cheese-laden bagels and far too much coffee, are willing to dissect and ponder the imponderable issues of our times. Drs. Stephen Vanner, John Rudan, Stephen Archer, and Michael Fitzpatrick are all highly accomplished examples of the doctors we need.

The "other world" that I was engaging in for the first time was that of publishing outside the realm of scientific papers and journals. This world, I found, is played by different, largely unwritten rules. Michael Levine, literary agent and much more, was able to encourage, guide, cajole, and maintain confidence when others would not.

I've bonded with Neil Seeman, as he's guided me through the editing process, over a shared passion to improve the lot of patients and physicians I've benefited greatly from the highly proficient and unfailingly patient editorial support of Sydney Druckman.

Finally, Michelle, who reads every word, hears every thought, and shares every emotion.

REFERENCES

Beagan, B. (2005). Everyday classism in medical school: Experiencing marginality and resistance. *Medical Education, 39*(8), 777–784.

Canadian Institute for Health Information. (n.d.). *A profile of physicians in Canada.* Retrieved from https://www.cihi.ca/en/a-profile-of-physicians-in-canada

Canadian Medical Association Journal. (2002). *CMAJ, 166*(8), 1029.

Canadian Medical Association. (n.d.). *Quick facts: Canada's physicians.* Retrieved from https://www.cma.ca/quick-facts-canadas-physicians

College of Family Physicians of Canada. (2018). *Family Medicine Professional Profile.* Mississauga, ON: College of Family Physicians of Canada.

Committee for Accreditation of Canadian Medical School Standards and Elements. (2023). *Standards and elements* (Standard 10, p. 18).

Commission on Generalism. (2011). *Guiding patients through complexity: Modern medical generalism.* London: Royal College of General Practitioners and the Health Foundation. Retrieved from http://www.rcgp.org.uk/policy/commissn_on_generalsm.aspx

Fowler, N., Oandasan, I., & Wyman, R. (Eds.). (2022). *Preparing Our Future Family Physicians: An Educational Prescription for Strengthening Health Care in Changing Times.* Mississauga, ON: College of Family Physicians of Canada.

Freidson, E. (1970). *Profession of Medicine: A Study of the Sociology of Applied Knowledge.* University of Chicago Press.

The Global Economy. (n.d.). *Doctors per 1,000 people by country.* Retrieved from https://www.theglobaleconomy.com/rankings/doctors_per_1000_people/

Greenhalgh, T., Seyan, K., & Boynton, P. (2004). "Not a university type": Focus group study of social class, ethnic, and sex differences in school pupils' perceptions about medical school. *BMJ, 328*(7455), 7455. Retrieved from https://doi.org/10.1136/bmj.328.7455.7455

Health Canada. (n.d.). *Canada Health Act*. Government of Canada. Retrieved from https://www.canada.ca/en/health-canada/services/health-care-system/canada-health-care-system-medicare/canada-health-act.html

Royal College of General Practitioners. (2012). *Medical Generalism: Why Expertise in Whole Person Medicine Matters*. London: Royal College of General Practitioners.

Sanfilippo, A. J., & Philpott, J. (2023, October 1). Family doctor shortage: Medical education can help address critical gaps, starting with a specialized program. *The Conversation*. Retrieved from https://theconversation.com/family-doctor-shortage-medical-education-can-help-address-critical-gaps-starting-with-a-specialized-program-169242

Statistics Canada. (2017). *2016 Census of Population: Age and sex release*. Retrieved from https://www12.statcan.gc.ca/census-recensement/2016/as-sa/98-200-x/2016004/98-200-x2016004-eng.cfm

Statistics Canada. (n.d.). *Table 13-10-0484-01 Life expectancy and other elements of the life table, Canada, all provinces except Prince Edward Island*. Retrieved from https://doi.org/10.25318/1310048401-eng

Steuart, J. (1767). *An Inquiry into the Principles of Political Economy* (Book 2, Chapter 2). Printed for A. Millar, and T. Cadell, in the Strand.